1 HABIT TO THRIVE IN A POST COVID WORLD

100 LIFE-CHANGING HABITS TO NAVIGATE THE POST-PANDEMIC WORLD FROM THE BEST-SELLING AUTHORS OF THE 1 HABIT BOOK SERIES

STEVEN SAMBLIS

FORBES RILEY

Edited by
BARB SWAN-WILSON

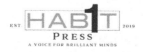

1 Habit to Pivot Your Life in a Post Covid World

By Steven Samblis, Forbes Riley and many Happy Achievers.

Published by 1 Habit Press, Inc.

Copyright © 2021 by 1 Habit Press, Inc. All rights reserved.

The publishers gratefully acknowledge the individuals that contributed to this book.

1 Habit™ and its Logo and Marks are trademarks of 1 Habit Press, Inc.

1 Habit Press, Inc.®

(310) 595-1260

30 North Gould Street

Suite 7616

Sheridan, WY 82801

www.1Habit.com

Copy Editor & Design: Steven Samblis

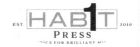

To my Daughters Lindsay and Kaitlyn

- Steven Samblis

To Ryker and Makenna, my twins, you are the wind beneath mommy's wings, and your love has allowed us all to fly!

This book is dedicated to YOU, whoever you are and wherever you are. I am YOU. A dreamer, a schemer, and TEAMER - We are in this together, and our rising tides shall lift all boats.

- Forbes Riley

FOREWORD

Welcome to 1 Habit to Pivot Your Life in a Post Covid World!

The first people I ever saw take a serious risk where my parents. In 1977, they bought a house well beyond their means, taking on a mortgage too expensive for them, during a time when interest rates were skyrocketing. Working constantly on the beautiful property overlooking the sea, they turned it into a home the envy of their friends and family. Years later, over dinner at a fancy restaurant, I asked my father – by then a Fortune 500 CFO – why they took on such a risk. He simply said, "We just thought things would get better." I learned a valuable axiom l that evening: Never underestimate your ability to overcome all obstacles with hard work and dedication.

It is a different era now. Like no time in the memories of most people alive today, the world around us has changed before our eyes. We are experiencing dynamic alterations in society, healthcare, economies, communication, technologies, attitudes, opportunities, and risks. Some have already become incredibly wealthy, some have discovered new callings, and some have seen their lives turned upside down. Learning to pivot the way we think and behave will be essential to survival, and, if you are aware enough, to prosper.

Post-war Europe went through such a time in the 1940s, '50s, and '60s. Many Europeans had to wait until the 1990s, almost 50 years after the end of WWII hostilities, to experience the freedoms the Allies said would be secured for the world if they were victorious. The lesson is that we must set out for our own success. We cannot depend on governments, companies, or religious institutions to come to our aid as we try to cope – or to pivot – in a post COVID world.

I am proud to say that Steve Samblis is a good friend. We frequently talk together about our careers and lifework, which are quite different from each other. Steve has spent most of his career in entertainment and the arts, while I have primarily been involved in finance and now am an executive at a growing restaurant company. As 2020 drew to a close, I called Steve. We talked about the books he had composed over the past 18 months, working with some of the most scholarly people across a wide range of professions. The purpose of my call was to see how he could work with some of these great minds and delve into their views on what was going on now to see how these leaders are looking to shift in light of the obvious change affecting us.

Beach, Florida. It was the early 80's. Cocoa Beach was a sleepy town where you could buy a charming home for under $50,000.00. Al was making a few million a year in commissions.

Al's office was right across from mine, so I every once in a while I would pop in his doorway and ask him how he became so successful, hoping to find the key. On one particular day, Al told me to sit down, watch, and listen. As he stood behind his desk, he picked up the phone and called a client, whom he later told me was a huge client but somewhat challenging to deal with. She always over-analyzed his recommendations, and by the time she was ready to pull the trigger, it was usually too late. "Mrs. Rooney, we have a terrific tax free bond yielding 8%, and I thought you would be interested." Al delivered the words, sat down, and shut up. It felt like an eternity went by as he sat silently on the phone, waiting for her response. "I have worked with you for many years, and during that time, you have missed out on incredible opportunities, which would have made you a great deal of money. This will be one of those. You have the money sitting in your Money Market, making a few points taxable. If you do not take this position, I am not doing my job and will no longer be able to be your Financial Advisor. I will pass your account on to somebody else." Al then stopped talking and waited. Another eternity went by until Al said. "Great, we will buy $200,000.00. I will place the order for you in the morning. Great decision. Talk to you soon."

I looked at Al stunned. "You were willing to throw away one of your biggest clients if she had said no?" Al went on to tell me that he had created a nightly Habit. Every evening at 6 pm, he looked at his book of 2000 clients and picked the five most difficult ones. He then called each one and gave them one shot to turn the relationship around, or he would dump them. He told me that this 1 Habit gave him a tremendous sense of peace. As it turned out, most clients just needed a little nudge to understand what a good position they were in having him manage their money. From that day forward, their attitudes and how they worked with him was dramatically improved.

As I left Al's office, I was inspired. I was motivated and worked hard, but motivation is just the thing that gets you started. It is Habits like Al's 6 pm calls that keep you going and drive you down the pathway to success.

Habits, once a part of you, are automatic. They don't drain your energy. They guide you along the right path to the life you want to live.

I went to my office, sat on my chair, and bounced up and went right back to Al's office. "Al, this is an amazing Habit, the 6 pm calls. However, I don't have 2000 clients. What one Habit could I make part of me that would get me to that 2000 client number?" Al took a moment and told me in a very matter of fact way. "Every night before you go home, map out your next day. If you have clients or prospects you will want to call tomorrow, make a list before you go home. If you have a trade ticket that you need to place in the morning, write it out before. Set yourself up for success every day by preparing the night before."

HOW TO MAKE A HABIT YOUR OWN

The Cycle of a Habit
All Habits follow a specific path

By Steven Samblis Creator of 1 Habit

The Habit

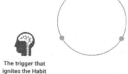

**The trigger that
ignites the Habit**

**The reward - All
Habits have
rewards attached**

Before we get into how to make a Habit your own, it is important to understand the cycle of a Habit. With this simple understanding, you will find it easier to make a Habit your own.

There is a cycle to all Habits. The cycle has three steps.

1st step: The Habit. It is the behavior you want to change, add, or remove.

2nd Step: The Reward. It is the payoff you get from the Habit.

3rd Step: The Trigger. It is the thing that makes you perform the Habit.

Keep this simple cycle in mind as you begin laying out your road map to making a Habit your own.

If you've ever tried to create a new Habit and have felt overwhelmed in the process of making even the slightest change, know that you're not alone. It's normal for emotions to come up when you're doing something new. It's also normal to want to QUIT and go back to your comfort zone, despite knowing those old Habits don't support your highest vision. As humans, we crave certainty. It makes us feel safe.

But safety doesn't always lead to success, and sometimes, risk is the best thing we can do to reap the rewards of leaning in and doing something different.

Realize that your *hands in the air* mentality when it comes to change won't serve you. Despite what you might think based on your old patterns or society's conditioning, you are capable of achieving anything you desire, and it starts with *choosing yourself first* and creating NEW Habits to fuel you forward, no matter what.

The Habits in all of our 1 Habit™ books have been carefully sourced by some of the most successful people to help you upgrade all areas of your life. The steps outlined below, as well as the inspiration laid out for you throughout these pages, *work if you work them.* So before you toss this book aside and let it collect dust, understand that this is not your typical "ra-ra" book. This is a book to challenge your beliefs, show you that what you want is on the other side of your fear (inaction) and that anything's possible when you commit to the process of change/upleveling.

If you think about your day to day routine, it's made up of Habits, right? And yes, some are better than others. That's okay! Change is possible, and you are more than capable. All of your current Habits, including the way you think, were created based on consistency - by YOU! So if you're feeling frustrated and wishing you could just (insert desire here), I am here to tell you that you absolutely can, and this book will help you get there... *faster.*

At this point, you might be evaluating what your current Habits are, and if you're not, I'm certain you will be by the end of this book. An important characteristic of a Habit is that it's automatic - you don't even think about it - so changing them takes conscious effort. Having awareness around how you spend your time and energy can be humbling, but it's necessary if you want to step into something greater. The truth is, we waste so much of our precious resources on things that don't move the needle forward because we've gotten so used to doing things a certain way.

The good news is, you have the power to change that at any time!

So how do you create new Habits that *stick?* Well, I've compiled a list of 30 steps that are not only proven to help you get started but also beneficial in supporting your long-term success. Before you read on, though, please understand that I am not asking you to do all of these things at once. I'm not crazy (and neither are you!). What I am inviting you to consider is that the way you're doing things right now isn't working (or you wouldn't be reading this book!). And more importantly, you can make positive changes in a short amount of time, starting small and gradually upgrading your daily Habits as they become a natural part of your routine.

After all, your morning coffee... your bath before bed... your need to answer every email as soon as it hits your inbox... the lack of time set aside for your workouts... even the route you take to and from work... all of these *Habits* were created *by you*, which means that only YOU have the power to change them.

Are you ready? Good! Let's get started.

1. **Set yourself up to win.** How many times have you told yourself you'd "start tomorrow" only to have tomorrow never come? I get it! Instead, focus on creating time and space and

understand what needs to be present for you to achieve the goal you've set for yourself.

2. Practice compassion. You are not perfect, and you never will be. That's a beautiful thing! So if things don't go exactly the way you envision, understand that there's a lesson there and honor where you're at, while acknowledging where you still have room to grow.

3. Be clear on your WHY. One of the biggest mistakes and reasons for failure is a lack of clarity around *why* you want to make the change in the first place. When your *why* is big enough, nothing can stop you - not even YOU!

4. Choose curiosity over judgment. Ugh, the infamous "judgment". Let's be honest; how well does that work for you? Instead, when you mess up (because you're human!), get curious. How could you have done it differently? How could you have shown up better? Who could you have asked for help? What needs to change to have a more positive result next time? Then rework your plan to support this new information.

5. Choose gratitude. *Gratitude turns what we have into enough.* Ever heard that saying? It's true! With everything and everyone that comes into your experience, give thanks for the opportunity to learn, grow, expand yourself. Remember to say THANK YOU for it all, and that includes having gratitude for yourself.

6. Stay consistent. The statement, *never skip a Monday,* could not be truer! When creating new Habits, it's important to keep your eye on the prize. If you want to get back to a regular workout routine, commit to moving your body *every single day* for 30 days. Skipping days while trying to create a new Habit will only make it harder to stick to. You'll notice that once you've completed those 30 days, your mind will be wired for movement (or whatever Habit you're implementing), and just like that, it's now part of your routine.

7. Find an accountability buddy. Everything is better with friends, right? Habits are no different, especially if it's a Habit that you want to create, but that feels reaaallllly hard to make happen. Grab your bestie and set up a check-in schedule, and make it fun!

8. Use visualization. Did you know there are now brain studies that show the power of our thoughts? In fact, it's been shown that our minds are capable of producing the same mental instructions as our actions.[1] Yea, how's that for some serious motivation! What we think, we become so think good thoughts and visualize them in the present moment as if they've already come to fruition. Add to that: *action,* and you'll be unstoppable.

9. Have a mantra. No, these aren't just for yogis. Think back to the *"Why"* you decided on (the reason you want to make this new Habit a reality). Create a statement or come up with a word that embodies the result you're working towards, or the way you want to feel in the process of instilling this new Habit. This can be an I AM statement (I AM capable... worthy... unstoppable...) or like I said, a single word like, HEALTHY. Whatever resonates for you, choose that. There is no right or wrong here.

10. **Notice your self-talk.** Every time a thought comes into your head that doesn't feel extra supportive, ask yourself: would I say this to my spouse... my child... my parents... my friends? If the answer is no, it's time to flip the script and create a more loving internal dialogue.

11. **Ask for support.** Yes, this might feel vulnerable. But just remember that people intrinsically want to help, so by asking for support, you are allowing others to give and getting in the practice of receiving. If this is uncomfortable for you, even better. Creating new Habits isn't meant to be easy; it's meant to challenge you and show you what you're made of, which is far more than you may realize.

12. **Identify your triggers.** Oh yes, the things that set us off and have us grabbing for the ice cream, or blowing our budget on a new pair of shoes! What (or who) are they? Write these down.

13. **Come up with positive responses to your triggers.** Now that you know what (or who) they are, how can you set yourself up to win if (when) they show up?

14. **Start small.** Small changes over time can make a massive impact. If you haven't worked out in years, saying you're going to run a marathon in a month probably isn't a great idea. Instead, can you commit to walking for at least 20 minutes each day and gradually increasing your time and intensity until you get where you want to go, physically? Decide what that looks like. Write it down.

15. **Choose ONE Habit to implement at a time.** I have a feeling you're ambitious, and you probably have a laundry list of things

you want to achieve. Good for you! But instead of trying to do all the things immediately, choose ONE thing. Getting a win under your belt releases dopamine in the brain (that feel-good chemical) and will inspire you to keep going!

16. Celebrate your wins. So now that you've got that dopamine swirling around CELEBRATE!! You did it, and that is amazing... YOU are amazing!

17. Keep a journal. It's okay if you're not a writer, the point of keeping track is to look back and see how far you've come. Writing down the emotions throughout the process can be an interesting gauge, and can provide a really beautiful space for growth and healing.

18. Be specific. Do you want to lose weight, or do you want to lose 10 pounds? The more specific you can get, the easier it will be to create a plan to set yourself up to win - and be able to recognize when success happens.

19. Create a plan. How are you going to achieve this? Who can help keep you on track? What needs to change so you can replace an old Habit with this new, more supportive one? Write it down.

20. Have a reward in mind for when you succeed! Have you been putting something on hold just waiting "until"? Now is the perfect time to allow yourself permission to indulge in the reward you've been pawning over. *"After I workout for 30 days in a row, I'm going to get myself those new shoes I've been eyeing to celebrate!"* Or maybe it's a trip you've wanted to take, or whatever it may be... let this be your permission slip to reward yourself for your hard work and celebrate the new Habit you just implemented into your life.

21. Believe that it's possible. Because it is! And you are far more capable than you may realize. *Whether you think you can or you think you can't, you're right. - Henry Ford*

22. Be so committed that nothing can stop you. Eye. On. The. Prize. That new Habit is not going to happen on its own! How bad do you want it? I hope you said something like, *more than anything.* What is not doing this costing you, your family, your life?

23. Record your affirmations (and use them!). Use the voice memo on your phone to record your mantra, an I AM statement, your "Why," something that PUMPS YOU UP and encourages you to stay the course. Listen as often as you need to in order to keep pushing, even when the going gets tough.

24. Share with a loved one. This is different than having someone do the work with you to reach your goal (that new Habit!). Simply stating your intention and plan to make it happen and asking others to support you in your efforts keeps the fire burning a little hotter. As humans, we want to know that people care and that they're proud of us. Letting your spouse or kids know that you're going to be making some changes can inspire the entire family to get on board. Pay it forward!

25. Get plenty of rest. We all know that feeling tired doesn't exactly lend well to motivation. Commit to getting uninterrupted sleep each night.

26. Drink a ton of water. Maybe don't drink a gallon of water before bed, but nourishing your cells with proper hydration not only helps you sleep better, it helps you stay energized and fueled during your day while helping to transport nutrients to your cells and wherever else they're needed. Water is the ultimate brainpower! And healthy brains make better decisions.

27. Nourish your mind, body, and soul. Surround yourself with people that will encourage and uplift you. These are the real angels on earth. We become the five people we spend the most time with, so make sure your circle supports the Habits you're looking to cultivate.

28. Avoid situations that would tempt you to "cheat" on yourself. If you know that joining everyone for a Happy Hour on Friday is going to cause you to indulge when you're committed to "clean eating without alcohol," do yourself a favor and skip it! There will be plenty more opportunities to partake in these things once you've gotten your Habits in check.

29. If you mess up, find the lesson, and keep moving forward. You are human, and you will mess up. Totally okay! Beating yourself up, harsh self criticism, and unwarranted negative self-judgment are not supportive, and just don't feel good. Let it go! And commit to doing better next time. Now, if you find that you use this mentality as an excuse to keep repeating mistakes, that's a different story. This is meant to forward you, not sabotage your progress.

30. Don't start without a plan. If you were driving cross-country, you'd probably pull out a map, right? The same goes for creating Habits. If you want to get from point A to point B with ease, see step 1 and set yourself up for success! Fail to plan, plan to fail. It's that simple.

So there you have it! Thirty steps to help you not only upgrade your Habits *but make them stick!* If you are serious about living your best life, your Habits are imperative to your success. Our intention for the 1 Habit™ series is to make this as easy as possible for you in the way of motivation, empowerment, and support.

You're an intelligent person, so I am confident you are fully aware that, as much as we'd love to make these changes for you, it's not possible. But our hope is that by laying out the foundation for you, you will not only begin to see how simple it can be - but also be inspired to get to work!

On behalf of myself and all of our contributors, WE BELIEVE IN YOU! Now get out there, create some new Habits, and achieve your dreams.

Resources:

https://www.psychologytoday.com/us/blog/flourish/200912/seeing-is-believing-the-power-visualization[1]

DEFINITION OF HABIT

Habit: A behavior pattern acquired by frequent repetition or physiologic exposure that shows itself in regularity or increased facility of performance.

- Merriam-Webster Dictionary

IMPORTANT NOTE - HOW TO USE THIS BOOK

1 Habit books are created to help you to find and instill new Habits that will change your life forever. These books are different from other "Self Help" books in the way they should be used.

Do not pick it up and read it from cover to cover.

The best way to use this book is as follows...

1. After you have read "How to Make a Habit Your Own", flip through the pages and let a Habit find you.
2. Decide if the Habit will enhance your life. If the answer is "Yes," go to step 3. (If not go back to step 1)
3. Follow the steps in the chapter "How to Make a Habit Your Own."

4. Once you have done so, and the Habit is a part of who you are, go back to step 1 and repeat.

Continue these steps, 1 Habit at a time, and you may change your life forever!

CONTENTS

1

GET BACK TO A DAILY SCHEDULE
STEVEN SAMBLIS

Why: This hit me like a ton of bricks recently. I was sitting at home and felt like taking a break. I thought to myself, "What day is it?" I have no idea. I had to look at my phone to see what day it was. This was a really uncomfortable realization. In my home office, I'm sitting at my desk, working on new books very successfully, but I had no idea what day it was. How dangerous is this for when this covid thing is over and we all back to regular schedules? How hard will it be to go back and treat a Friday like a Friday? That may be an easy one. But what about treating Wednesday like a Wednesday. We had all these built-in alarm bells in life that kept us on course and pace, and we ran our race through the week. Now that is all gone, and the result is startling.

Now, don't get me wrong. I killed it during covid. But little by little, days morphed into each other. It made it easy to start binge-watching Cobra Kia at noon on a Tuesday. After all, there was no World "work clock" that we were all adhering to anymore.

One day when I got around to taking a shower, I changed out of my sweats and t-short to a brand new pair of sweats and a t-shirt.

This was all happening while new authors were coming in, and we were spitting out one best-selling book after another.

Well, I realized that this was not a sustainable life path and got back to the clock. I created routines. I planned my days and thought about what day each day was. I celebrated Friday! I had not done this in almost a year.

The best way to do this create the Habit of putting yourself back on a clock. Think about each day and treat each one differently. Schedule breaks. Schedule luck, dinner, date nights.

This small Habit will refocus you and get you in sync for, as Ayn Rand would say -- When the World's engine starts up again.

Time to prepare to jump on board.

THE UN-HABIT: FORGETTING TO DRESS FOR SUCCESS

Why: The one great thing and the un-great thing about having a set schedule and going to an office was you would dress for success.

Here is what happens when you dress up and look in the mirror; you feel great. Even if you are not leaving the house, you feel better. All over us bought more sweat pants and t-shirts to re-dress our new world. That was nice and comfy for a few months, but it sucked the soul and pride out of us in the process.

It is time to get back to looking good and feels good as a result.

This is such an easy habit to break. Even though many of us will still be working from home when this is over (Which I have done for years and love), we need to take the time in the morning to get back to the ritual of preparing ourselves for the day ahead. We need to do this by showering, putting on proper clothes that you would be proud to wear to any meeting, and getting back to the business of being a rock star in our industries!

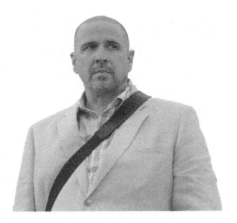

ABOUT STEVE: I am the creator of the bestselling 1 Habit book series, published by 1 Habit press, a vertically integrated media company focusing on the development of human potential.

2

EMBRACE TECHNOLOGY
FORBES RILEY

Why: The year was 1997, Hotmail just launched, and my dad, a skilled mechanic, engineer, and inventor, threw up his hands in frustration and said, "This internet stuff will never catch on, too complicated."

He died shortly after that at just 70. Fast forward not more than 20 years, and technology is moving faster than our imaginations can keep up with. The question is, How do we keep up?"

Well, if you don't continue to change, pivot, and adapt, you will end up disappearing like the giant companies that we all believed would last forever, Radio Shack, Kodak, and Blockbuster. They also looked at new technology and new ways of thinking and shook their head or threw their hands up and said, "Oh, it just won't last."

I started hearing people say that about COVID, "I can't wait for things to go back to normal."

It turns out things never go back; they only move forward. And a new normal means that you must keep an open mind and master the Habit of embracing new technology. And like they say about how you eat an elephant, one bite at a time. Go slow as there is a lot to digest, but learn a little bit daily, and in no time, you will be astounded at how your daily life will improve and be made more relevant. Dad, I miss you so much; your stubbornness inspired me, a hunger and a thirst and a need to keep current. And I do wish you could see all the cool things we can do today.

#1 Zoom: Imagine no longer having to get on a plane and travel across the country to take an in-person meeting? Today I meet with students and clients worldwide; thanks to Zoom, it almost feels like we are sitting at the same table. As a pre-pandemic person who traveled up to 200 days a year, I have saved money, precious time, and my sanity! I even celebrated my birthday in a Zoom Meeting room and partied with family and friends, some of who I hadn't seen in years, AND they all got to meet each other. I host fitness classes and seminars all from the comfort of my living room, and I urge you to enjoy all the new improvements the platform has made, from green screen technology to break-out private meeting rooms.

#2 Canva: No longer do I have to wait a week for my graphic artists to get back to me to change a font or create a new banner for an ad. I find myself in Canva almost every day, creating Facebook posts or workbooks, vision boards, to greeting cards.

Make it a habit to express your creativity again and have it downloadable in just seconds.

#3 www.Forbes360.com: This is one of my go-to daily technologies that has allowed me to get my message out there, build an active email list, and connect with people in a truly meaningful way. In the old days, I hired WebMasters to build pages, and I was always so frustrated with their lack of commitment - I wasted so much time and money. Now in under an hour, I can do it. There are so many things that I use in the new technology. And lastly, understand how to create your own web page and sales funnel quickly to promote your message.

So smile and move forward with a habit of levelling up your tech!

THE UN-HABIT: STOP SITTING STILL

Why: When COVID hit gyms shut down, and warned to stay at home, not go out and shelter in place. For a moment, my world collapsed.

I enjoy going to the gym, doing Pilates, roller skating, paddle boarding, dancing, long walks after a long day, and moving around every single day. That is what I do as a healthy lifestyle expert and what my mentor Fitness Guru, Jack Lalanne instilled in me. He also preached until he was 96 that you need to get 20 minutes daily of "safe sun" from sitting outside to get sunshine; that's how your body produces vitamin D, an essential vitamin your body produces only from sunlight to aid in fighting off infection. April 2020, and we're stuck inside our homes, fearing to go outside with no fresh air and no sunlight. Suddenly there seemed to be a great depression in the air.

We need to move around, not sit still.

As the months wore on, I prepared to fight back! Turns out I had created an amazing solution to an impossible dilemma. How do you move and stay fit inside while sitting at your desk on endless Zoom calls? You SpinGym! The simple handheld fitness product based on a 2000-year-old Chinese toy called a Button and String. According to a Stanford Study, this compact marvel rotates at over 125,000 PRM and, when used for 2 minutes, burns and ignites every muscle in your upper body. Now it's fair to be skeptical, but all you need to do is try it and experience it once, and you'll be hooked.

In May 2020, I began teaching free daily classes on Zoom, and I watched how the attitude and energy of everyone onboard just blossomed.

It quickly became apparent that moving daily, breaking a sweat, and the companionship of a group class was, in fact, an antidote to the depression and frustration that had been building in so many of us.

Now you may be asking, "Do I need a SpinGym to feel better, or will yoga, resistance bands, or dumbbells do the trick?"

Well, If you've never touched a SpinGym, you have no idea how effective and intense the resistance can be. To be clear, I did not invent the technology behind SpinGym, but I did harness it into a product we all can benefit from. With all my heart, I believe that using this ancient inspired apparatus can change your state of mind, give you a boost of energy, and make you break a sweat in just a few minutes. You feel it immediately as it vibrates through your body and instantly activates almost every muscle in your upper body. When using it for just one song on your playlist, your arms are on fire, your shoulders ignite, your abs engaged, and your core is doing what it's supposed to do - support your spine.

So, my Habit is to move daily, but not just move. You need to break a sweat, elevate your heart rate, and have fun. Do I sound like a commercial for SpinGym? Perhaps, but if I don't, you would never hear about this, and that would be a shame. I found a powerful and healing solution for the mind, body, and spirit, so why not share it.

To date, on home shopping channels around the globe, I've sold 2.2 million, but odds are you haven't heard of it as I haven't focused on the marketing. I'm telling you now because we all must focus on our health during this post-covid time, and it would be a shame if you haven't yet experienced what all the buzz is all about.

So, If you're like me and you spend too much time sitting on zoom calls, my Habit is that you do SpinGym for 60 seconds, once every hour. For the tiny investment of time, everyone reports being happier, feeling energized, and several have lost upwards of 30 pounds in this past year alone.

The year has taught us to pivot and embrace a new normal.

An unexpected side effect and serious downsides of the COVID lockdown is a looming level of depression and feeling lost. If you compound that with eating processed food, indulging too much in sweets, pasta, pizza, and candy, AND you do not move your body, it will take a negative toll on your overall health.

We must fight back, and one solution is to make a Habit of Daily SpinGym. Please don't hesitate to reach out to me with any comments or questions. As you're reading this, my team and I offer a free seven day Jump Start your Fitness challenge. The links can all be found at www.ForbesRiley.com

My goal is to motivate and inspire you to be your very best. Start getting fit today or a year from now, you will wish you did.

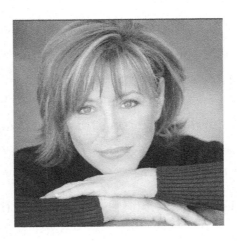

About Forbes: Forbes Riley mesmerizes audiences with her authentic, inspirational style that is second to none. Often referred to when she hosts tv shows and speaks on stage, as Oprah meets Tony Robbins, in the unique way she transports, transforms, and transfixes audiences all around the world.

As one of the pioneers behind the As Seen on TV infomercial phenomenon, Forbes Riley has hosted 180+ infomercials and guested on QVC/HSN generating more than $2.5 billion in global sales.

Her goal today, post-Covid it to inspire and motivate people to achieve their dreams and beyond through group coaching www.PitchSecretsMasterClass.com

Her vast and diverse career has allowed her to experience the best and worst of what life has to offer. As the co-author of several one habit books from entrepreneurial success to thriving home office and post COVID Habits, she is honored and blessed to work with some of the best, from her students and clients to co-authors and mentors.

Her personal motto: You may only live once, but if you do it right. Once is enough.

3

MULTIPLY RESULTS BY FOCUSING ON PEOPLE

MARIO ELSNER

Why: Out of necessity, I had to live alone from an incredibly young age, 15 years, without guidance and support, I had to learn to succeed in life. I had to make up for all my shortcomings as well as I could. The road was hard, but I learned that to achieve extraordinary results and cope with the worst of situations, the solution was to surround myself with talented people either to receive knowledge or create teams that would potentiate my results. Alone, maybe I could achieve them, but I would burn out. Not having the freedom to jump into my dreams just gave me baby steps toward them.

As I focus on people, I move from being alone to having ten families, those of my friends, from being a good salesman, to outperform all the sales records, assembling a team that applied my methodologies in their day to day, generating an automated system, in which I was investing time on guidance, not in doing everything.

To be honest, this requires patience and a tremendous recruiting system for the best talent. But right now, I can manage a million-dollar company and spend lots of time helping other people to achieve their goals, using today's tools that during Covid19 has become a reality, to build communities globally.

Teams, affiliates & Communities DO NOT add up; they Multiply Reach and results.

So, from those days, I understood that my most significant investment should be behind people. There is no way to make a difference in life; if you think you will achieve it alone, you must use others' strengths and knowledge. My life is based on finding, training, and consolidating multi-functional teams that expand the established limits, always breaking the Status Quo. There are no limits or Boundaries.

Imagine that you implement the Uber system in your life; you use a leverage effect to have a global footprint. That is what happens when your life purpose is based on building around people.

THE UN-HABIT: TRYING TO DO EVERYTHING ALONE

Why: We believe that no one does a job better than ourselves. If we do not drive the ship, it will not get to safety. But this is simply a story we tell ourselves to feel important.

What is a reality is that there will be no one like us, but that doesn't mean there are no better people than us in other skills. Having the humility to accept our limitations is the first step in becoming leaders and not doers. Do not think on being a Captain; work on becoming a fleet admiral.

There is a big difference between a Solo entrepreneur and a business owner. While it would not be the same way of doing things, your way, the speed, and results can be outstanding if you can surround yourself with talented people and build a multi-functional team.

What is the use of getting to your objectives, burnout? Part of the process of becoming successful in live and achieve extraordinary goals is enjoying the journey.

So, think every day, which tasks you can delegate to focus on making a difference and getting to your life purpose faster.

YOU ARE NOT ALONE in this world

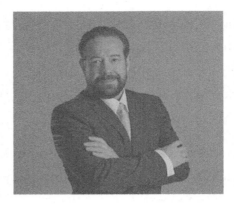

ABOUT MARIO: Mario Elsner is on a mission to create a movement to change the world, helping others achieve their goals using multi-functional teams & performance indicators. With more than 20 years in Global FMCG companies with international experience in Latin America, Mario founded an online platform & community for entrepreneurs & Business Owners to learn about major corporate systems to implement in their lives to become successful in generating an impact.

With his methodologies & mentorship programs, you will understand and execute key drives to explode your company in 10X. Just see him as Mr. Miyagi of the business; he teaches not only the what, but the why and the how.

4

INVEST IN YOU

SALLY GREEN

hy: To "pivot" in a post-Covid world, I invite you to consider an investment in yourself. We must be physically, emotionally, and spiritually fit to move forward, or else we will stay stuck and feel overwhelmed. During the quarantine of 2020, I decided that it was time to invest in myself, something I hadn't done in years. I began taking online courses, attending workshops, reading books, exercising, and eating healthier. I had a complete transformation, and I do not plan to ever go back to my pre-Covid me.

Physical Investment: Your body has remarkable superpowers. When you stop doing what is causing your body damage, it begins healing itself more quickly than you ever thought possible. As far as the food you're consuming, it is time to get back to nature. Start by preparing and cooking your foods and step away from processed, sugary, and salty meals and snacks.

You can do some things to invest in your physical health, learn to cook new dishes, research on how to make your favorite recipes healthier, and start an exercise regimen.

Mental/Emotional Investment: To get things done in a post-covid world, you need to be mentally and emotionally strong. Connecting with other people, building strong relationships, and cultivating a positive self-image all help build resilience. There are many tools to improve your mental health. Taking time to plan your day, visualizing positive outcomes to challenges, and caring for a pet, are just a few approaches you could use. Another helpful technique for growing a healthy mindset is to find a hobby or passion that makes you happy. I enjoy painting, but for others, it may be music or knitting or woodworking. Find something that brings you joy. Invest in a hobby and schedule activities that will improve your mental health.

Spiritual Investment: One of the best ways to grow spiritually is to take a walk in nature. While on your walk, notice the smells, sounds, and feelings you get while being outside. Years ago, I discovered a meditation and visualization technique that has helped me immensely. It requires you to take time each day to be still, meditate and visualize. Meditation helps reduce worry and anxiety. It is something I highly recommend. Other ways to grow spiritually include:

• Reading uplifting books

• Listening to inspirational speakers

• Attending local faith services

- Journaling

- Making a gratitude list

- Performing acts of service

- Taking yoga classes

Investing in you is something that no one can ever take away. Learning, reading, listening, and taking action can lead to new opportunities and long-term positive change. It may not be easy, but it will be worth it. Having a healthy mind, body, and spirit will enhance your life.

THE UN-HABIT: TURN OFF THE TELEVISION

Why: Nobody at the end of their life says, I wish I had watched more television. One thing Covid taught me is that life is short. I realized that watching TV created anxiety, and while I continue to watch movies and sports, I stopped watching everything else. Because of this, I was able to get more done and feel better. One of the most obvious benefits was time. I have been using the time to read, take online courses, exercise, and focus on my hobby as an acrylic and watercolor artist. In 2020, I created over 50 paintings while listening to music and setting up my paint area instead of watching nightly sitcoms.

Another benefit of stepping away from the daily habit of television watching is reducing the amount of stress and anxiety associated with living in a Covid and post-Covid world. I noticed a change in my attitude and anxiety levels right away. Most of the news stations are alarming and sensationalist.

Choosing to follow good sources of news and information has helped me feel less stressed. And by not listening to all the hype and researching the facts myself, I was less afraid.

I also feel that I have developed a deeper sense of my purpose and goals. I was hypnotized, zoned out, and living in a make-believe world while the real world around me kept spinning. Instead of dealing with my challenges and setbacks, I was wasting time being distracted by what I was watching. Although television is an escape, I realized it was affecting my health.

Shutting off the boob-tube has made me healthier. I am up moving around more. I have more energy; my relationships are better; my family has had many engaging and wonderful conversations. I have spent more time on the telephone checking in with people and interacting on FaceTime and zoom calls this year than I ever have before. I am enjoying cultivating new relationships and learning more about my family and friends.

Try shutting off the television and see what you can accomplish!

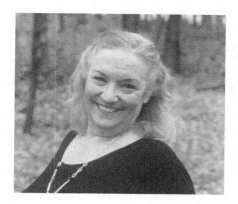

ABOUT SALLY: Sally Green lives in Connecticut with her husband Billy, and her daughter Amanda. As a successful small business owner, she was asked to contribute to the book, "1 Habit for Entrepreneurial Success". Her experience as an Inspirational speaker, Christian educator, and Woman's Bible Study leader spans over 30 years. Sally is a spiritual growth coach and teaches a meditation and visualization technique in her "Habits for Faith" program. She has written an inspirational book of poetry and two bible studies.

5

PAYING ATTENTION TO MONEY AND ME

BARB SWAN-WILSON

Why: As a young adult, the advice to use my brains, not my brawn, was often given to me. Did I listen? Hmm, not so much! I loved being physical, play hard, work hard. I was a smart kid. At 18 years old, I invested in my retirement but was swindled out of it by my controlling penny-pinching husband.

With life experience, we do become wiser, and our wealth is directly related to our health. A near-death illness shook my world, opened my eyes, and broadened my horizons. I lost almost everything, my confidence, business, identity, support network, retirement funds (declared bankruptcy), and lost my beloved connection with my 1,000s of customers.

Incredible amounts of good came from that illness (look for the silver lining in all things that appear bad.) That is not what my Habit is about.

My eyes and mind are now open to accept all things that will serve me well in my life. My health is my most important asset, and I am learning to take better care of myself. I've tried all kinds of health products, and yes, many of them worked wonders, but they are quite expensive for someone who is starting over after leaving their husband. I had to find a way to afford these life-enhancing products. For years I joined various companies, used and sold the products but never found the perfect fit for me; until 2020.

Our lives all changed in 2020, as did mine, but mine was in such a fantastic way. We launched Healthy Mugs, a family business that creates memory mugs (with personalized messages), and we connect people with an affordable, highly nutritious, good for you, energy drink. This powdered food drink mixed with 2 oz of mango juice is my Elixir of life, my magic mango mix!

I do something great for my health every morning. My Habit is to drink my mango elixir. After a few weeks of consuming this, something magical happened; my lower back pain dropped off the chart. It had me hooked, I loved the taste, and it is affordable. I don't always eat the best, so I need nutrition and energy; this has me covered—250% of my vitamin D, 100% of my C, and 1,600% of my B12, to list only three of 120 botanicals, minerals, and antioxidants.

My Habit improves my health, my mental clarity, and my wealth. It is easy on my bank account when I buy it, and it is one of several of my income streams.

THE UN-HABIT: THINKING THE DREAM HAS VANISHED

W**HY**: I thought I lost my dreams; my decorating center, children, fairy tale marriage, fishing every weekend, and spending lots of time with friends and family. What is there to live for? What is my purpose?

Depression is a stealthy adversary and creeps into the crevices of our minds. As optimistic as I am, it still has reared its ugly head several times in my life. I win the battle every time now; my mindset and my magic mango mix are my armor. Your mindset is a choice, and for me, it is the most powerful weapon we have.

Remarried and unhappy. Why? Nothing on my dream list was coming true. I am isolated in my marriage because my spouse suffers from PTSD (Post Traumatic Stress Disorder) and isolated in my location (no neighbors for a kilometer). My family and friends live 10 hours away.

Covid strikes another blow, lockdowns! As an isolated extrovert living in lockdown, I wasn't a happy camper. I was ready to throw in the towel and move in with my parents. I kept saying to myself, what about me? I matter too! I deserve to be happy. I was getting depressed, and I knew it.

Then along came Zoom meetings, networking, and people, glorious connections with people—a silver lining.

Forbes Riley reminded me that we get what we tolerate, and I couldn't tolerate an unhappy life anymore!

So I changed my mindset, and I shared how I felt. I wasn't willing to throw away 12 years of marriage. I changed how I thought and the messages that played in my head. I ran thoughts of our first years together, our plans, our dreams, how we would change the world and grow old together. Those renewed thoughts sparked a change in both of us.

My dreams will live on, adjusted to suit a higher purpose of the divine spirit of the universe. The new path is leading me to achieve significantly larger goals on multiple levels.

Covid lockdowns have created hundreds of thousands of people who now have PTSD. My dreams have shifted into ways to help the world recover from the trauma of abuse brought on by family members who suffer PTSD.

My Habit is to course correct when needed, and shift my mindset.

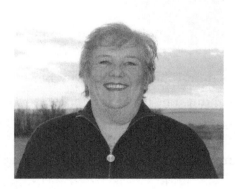

About Barb: An artisan wordsmith who crafts unique messages of your memories and preserves them in a chapter in a 1Habit book or wrapped with love around a coffee mug.

Barb Swan-Wilson is the co-founder of Healthy Mugs, providing you with motivational messages on mugs and drinkware, inspiring friends, family, coworkers, and your clients to take a moment and HugAMug to enjoy a few minutes of peace.

Healthy Mugs donates to an (OSI) Occupational Stress Injury group (another name for PTSD) and plans to collaborate in creating a not-for-profit foundation to support family members with the costs of counselling.

Barb likes to help you stay happy, healthy, and connected with cheerful ideas, nutritional energy drinks, and help you put checkmarks beside bucket list wishes.

With diverse life experiences from a tradesperson, kitchen design trainer, decorating center owner, bowling alley proprietor, sales director, and editor, Barb brings a wealth of knowledge and understanding to the conversation.

6

CREATE AND MAINTAIN YOUR PERSONAL DEVELOPMENT PLAN

ALAN FLEMING

Why: This is your blueprint for success in a post-Covid world.

The Covid pandemic will have an enormous impact on our health and livelihoods for many years to come. Its aftermath will undoubtedly influence the way we work, shop, interact, and study in the future. Business owners, for example, had to adapt swiftly to remote working strategies to survive the pandemic. These flexible arrangements became very popular in the United Kingdom, and by April 2020, approximately 49% of adults worked from home due to the outbreak.

The pandemic allowed many employees time to assess their career prospects and opportunities. According to Aviva (UK), more than half of UK workers planned to make changes to their careers in the following year. In both scenarios, the best candidates quickly recognized that the labour market was in a state of flux and reacted accordingly. They also made it a habit to regularly maintain their personal development plan, keeping their CVs up to date, and finding ways to maximize their potential in a competitive marketplace.

A personal development plan is one of the most important documents that you need to prepare to survive in a volatile post-Covid world. While many individuals embrace personal development as a lifelong self-improvement process, most fail to create an action plan to track and monitor their strengths and weaknesses in key aspects of their life. These include their knowledge, skills, education, career, wealth, health, spiritual wellbeing, and aspirations, to name a few.

Personal development plan templates are readily available on the internet, and you can customize the documents to meet your particular requirements. It's important to remember that your plan is a living document and reflects your unique set of circumstances.

Preparing a personal development plan will allow you to:-

• set goals and consider what you want to achieve personally or during your career,

• formulate an action plan to keep you focused on your goals or objectives in the short, medium, or long-term,

- undertake a self-assessment to gain awareness about where you are now, where you want to be in the future and how you plan to get there,

- embark on a journey of self-discovery to identify your strengths and weaknesses across the critical aspects of your life,

- keep records about what you have achieved to date, and

- to evaluate and review important stages in your development over time.

The Covid pandemic and impact on the global economy will make it more difficult for job seekers to climb the career ladder. Investing time in your personal development plan will be crucial when competing against other candidates in a highly competitive labour market.

THE UN-HABIT: OVERCOME PROCRASTINATION TO SUCCEED

Why: "I'm taking care of my procrastination issues; just you wait and see."

Procrastination is the action of delaying or postponing something. It was derived from the Latin word *procrastinatus*, which evolved from the prefix *pro-*, meaning *"forward"* and *crastinus*, meaning *"of tomorrow."* [Karen K. Kirst-Ashman; Grafton H. Hull, Jr. (2016)]. In other words, put things off until tomorrow.

It was easy to fall into the trap of binge-watching movies, television shows, sport, and documentaries during the global pandemic. Many families turned to Netflix, Now TV, Amazon, and Apple TV to distract themselves during the lockdown. They missed a golden opportunity to work on their skills and personal development during that time. Instead, most would procrastinate about what they wanted to achieve during their time at home, rather than engaging themselves in some of the growing lists of online courses available on the internet.

There was a significant rise in the number of distance learning courses created during the pandemic as training providers switched from face-to-face teaching in the classroom to online education using digital platforms. According to Research and Markets, the global online education market is forecast to reach US$320bn by 2025.

Engaging in distance learning does not always cost money. For example, YouTube delivers over a billion views of learning-related video content every day and mostly free of charge through its educational channels. Microsoft also offers free, customizable product training through its Microsoft 365 learning pathways; it provides various learning paths and modules via its Microsoft Learn portal. Students can sit for their examinations from the comfort of their home for a relatively small fee.

Certain training providers offer their courses through a monthly subscription model. For example, LinkedIn Learning offers over five thousand courses within its online educational platform, and most include certifications as part of the fee structure.

Universities and colleges offer distance learning and online courses as an alternative route to studying for a degree. It also gives their students the flexibility of studying from anywhere in the world. Leading universities such as Harvard, Oxford, and Cambridge have partnered with third-party platform providers to make their executive and professional education courses accessible to a global audience.

The options for learning and personal development continue to grow, and many excellent courses are now accessible from our homes. If you suffer from procrastination, enrolling and completing your first course will help you overcome your fears.

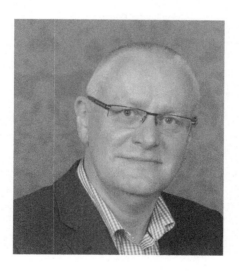

About Alan: Alan Fleming, is a Project Manager, with a strong track record in on-time project delivery and expertise working with Microsoft Dynamics CRM and ERP solutions. When you are struggling with a new piece of technology that they promised would connect seamlessly, who do you reach out to for help? Wouldn't it be nice in this ever-changing world of high-tech gadgets and software to have a quick and easy to understand project plan at your fingertips? When you need computer solutions, we are there to help you solve your problems!

7

SMILE, BE GRATEFUL, ENJOY L.I.F.E.
MARTIN SALAMA

Why: In the Covid world we're living in today, simple acts like smiling, especially in public, are not happening much. It seems we're all getting too deep within ourselves and allowing the world to negatively affect us instead of us positively affecting the world, even if it's one person at a time. The first person you can effect change in is yourself! That's right — it starts with you. Here's your PIVOT in a Post-Covid World.

One of my favorite authors, Genevieve Davis, writes, "The world is as you see it." Simply put, if you see the world as a positive, wonderful place full of opportunities, then that is what the world will present to you.

Imagine if you went around and smiled all the time. People would want to be with you; they would want what you have, what you know! It doesn't cost anything to smile at someone. I try my best to do it as much as possible. I have often been told that I smile a lot and look happy. Until recently, I would thank the person and not pay much attention to it. But lately, I've been noticing it more. I often thank them and say I've come to truly appreciate my life and everything in it. I share with them that I have implemented a new mindset of happiness and joy, even when things aren't going well, and finish by telling them about my acronym mantra — L.I.F.E. and my attitude to "Live Incredibly Full Everyday." It's that positive mindset shift that makes all the difference in the world.

Before, when people asked how I was, I would answer that I had no complaints. Then I would add that even if I had complaints, no one cared. There was an underlying message that I was I conveying, a message of apathy and discontent. It served no one, not myself or the person I was talking to. Instead, I decided to smile, say everything is wonderful, and mean it.

People can tell when you're sincere and when you "fake to make it," so be sincere. The cashier in the grocery store, the delivery person, the plumber, and the gas station attendant will appreciate it, and you might just make their day. Often when I interact with people, I try to get them to smile or laugh. When they laugh, I say I'm working on filling my quota of making people laugh for the day. It usually gets them to laugh more. Who knows, maybe they'll Pay It Forward!

HAB1T™

THE UN-HABIT: FROWN, BE SAD, COMPLAIN, AND DO NOTHING ABOUT IT.

WHY: You never know how what you say or do will affect someone. This goes both ways. Imagine if you walked around all day with a scowl on your face; you were dejected and unpleasant to everyone around you. You'd be miserable, but, just as important, your attitude would negatively affect the people around you. You would give off and attract complaints, and no one would want to be with you. Your attitude is infectious when you complain, are short with someone, or groan. The people around you will feel it. Let's go back to the Genevieve Davis quote, "The world is as you see it." In this scenario, if you see the world as a negative, unhappy place with nothing to offer, then that is what you'll get from it. Most people have heard of "The Law of Attraction." At its simplest, it means what you put out is what you attract. There is a lot more to it, and it's far from simple. However, in this example, it can be as simple as that. Like Energy Attracts Like Energy.

Think about the time of Covid and the attitude that's been permeating the world. Other than the occasional feel-good story that might put a temporary smile on your face, it's been dreary, hopeless, and downright sad out there. And, let's face it, the effect of these stories is temporary because, at the end of the day, it's probably not a feel-good story that impacts you or your daily life.

So how is all this negativity serving you? I'm sure the answer is not well. Why is that? It's because you're letting it affect you!

You've allowed all the bad news around you to create a bad habit of complaining, sadness, and depression in so many people. The adage of "it's not what happens to you, it's how you react or respond to what's happening" is more important now than ever. So why not change that habit of negativity, complaining, and what happens to you. Make your new habit one of positivity, gratitude, and response of acceptance and finding the good in everything that comes your way.

Adopt my acronym mantra and remember to Enjoy L.I.F.E. and Live Incredibly Full Everyday!

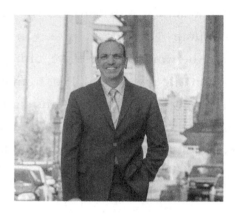

About Martin: Hi, my name is Martin Salama. I'm known as the Architect of The Warriors L.I.F.E. Code. I specialize in helping people frustrated in their life quickly shift their mindset to *UNCOVER* their greatness so they can live their true potential and enjoy LIFE!

An example of what I've achieved is a client like Roberta, who lost her 6-figure job due to COVID and came to me depressed and felt very lost. Within a short time, she told me she had "direction, focus, and a renewed energy around all the possibilities I could pursue... and getting back on track to enjoy LIFE!"

The key to my success is, I've mastered the ability to Live Incredibly Full Everyday! Which I turned into the acronym LIFE and created the Warriors L.I.F.E. Code coaching program.

8

WEAR SOMETHING DIFFERENT DAILY

INGA GOODMAN

Why: Do you have a favorite food? I couldn't imagine spending my life without chocolate, coconut, and green tea ... seriously, I've tried. Does it mean that I have those foods for breakfast, lunch, and dinner every day? Of course not! If your favorite food is pizza, it doesn't mean you want to have it for dinner three nights in a row. Eventually, anyone will become tired of, if not displeased with, the same eats.

There is a good reason that there are a million different kinds of coffee beans, beer and wine, bread, ice cream, and cake recipes in addition to potato chips that come with jalapeno, cheddar cheese, olive oil, sea salt, vinegar (you name it) exist. Yet every year, chefs from all over the world create new dishes and flavor combinations, while flavor chemists continue designing the next amuse-bouche to delight consumers.

Our minds, like our bodies, naturally require diversity. Even slight changes have a positive effect on peoples' mindset, mood, relationships, productivity, and creativity, whether it is a new set of towels in your bathroom, wallpaper, furniture arrangement, new playlist, or a simple change of scenery. "If you do not create change, change will create you."

Although humans are; creatures of habit, allowing diversity in one's life and breaking down routines once in a while brings positive mental, emotional and physical changes. Events such as an unexpected surprise or the natural change of seasons can boost your emotional state.

Clothes are no exception! In fact, switching what you wear is the quickest and easiest impactful way to bring that needed change to your daily grind, both externally and internally, by stimulating your eye and refreshing your mind. Even more so when you lack an opportunity to bring any other changes to life or you are simply forced to spend most of your time in the same place and can't get out, wearing a new outfit is a chance to start fresh every day despite any other circumstances.

As a fashion designer and stylist, I've strongly promoted the idea of embracing change through changing the look of your clothing. I experience instant and positive effects when I change my outfit. My clients constantly provide me with glowing reports on how a new outfit brings a mindset shift and a productivity boost to them as well.

The implication here is not a style makeover; rather, the notion is to utilize every single option already in your closet, literally wear a different piece of clothing, and use new combinations within your wardrobe daily!

Not only will you look and feel different every time you get dressed but picking out a different piece of clothing to wear each day of the week, it's also a keen way to get rid of that guilt that many of us feel while looking at all the unworn clothes in our closets. Two birds with one stone, bam!

THE UN-HABIT: WEARING PJs AROUND THE CLOCK!

Why: You heard me right! Ditch PJs out of your day and leave them where they truly belong – in your bedroom. The reason is structure; something all pajamas are lacking! It's fascinating how the absence of structure in your clothing directly translates into an absence of structure in your thoughts and, by extension, your actions. Blame your subconscious!

Your subconscious, your brain, and your actions are all closely related. Each time we take a certain action, we cause our subconscious to respond by sending specific signals to your brain, signals responsible for our further actions. The subconscious's role is to keep you safe, and each time it encounters an unfamiliar or atypical situation in your routine, it causes your brain to 'freak out'.

Big lottery winners are a well-documented example of this ... statistics show that over seventy percent of all people who win big in the lottery become broke within the first year! Why? They haven't had any experience managing large amounts of money; their subconscious doesn't know what to do with the new experience and sees this as a threat.

Imagine what kind of messages your brain will receive if you decide to bungee jump or ride in a rodeo without any prior training. How is your subconscious going to react? Translate that into staying in your PJs all day; your subconscious mind says "day off," but it is a workday. I'd rather go to bed dressed as casual chic than stay in my sleepwear all day.

There is a good reason that we wear workout attire to the gym, not to a business meeting, uniform to school or office, gowns and tuxedos to events, and it's not always about convenience.

You are not on a mission in your yoga pants and a tank top. You may be on the way to your next yoga session, but you are not on a mission. These extra couple of minutes that you spend in the morning changing out of your loose, shapeless sleeping set with stretched out knees into your superhero suit go a long way!

Blame your subconscious!

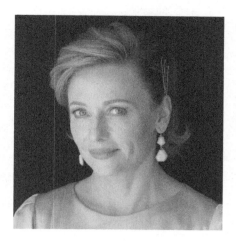

ABOUT INGA: Do you ever wish you could live a better life? I can assure you that it's possible just by improving your style! I'm a fashion designer who for years has been igniting women to live up to their fullest potential through fashion. Would you like to see how my designs can transform your life?

9

NEVER STOP ASKING QUESTIONS
DR. MANON BOLLIGER

Why: They say the quality of the question informs the quality of the answer.

Be comfortable with not knowing an answer. Rather, stay open and curious, and do your own research to find the answers you seek.

In today's society, we are bombarded with multiple opinions, points of view, and facts from multiple sources, and it is up to us as individuals to find our truth within the storm of information.

In a world where freedom of speech and the sharing of different points of view or opinion are being threatened due to its being classified as 'fake news', we need to ensure that we have the basis on which to establish our own perspective.

Asking questions of our governments, media, scientists, social outlets, and more, will allow you to carve out your path of truth within a society that suppresses information on the basis of protection.

2021 is the year to discover radical self-responsibility and freedom of choice. If there is a part of you that prefers to be a follower or is more comfortable to belong to the "herd" around you, then you must ensure that the herd is moving in the direction you intend to go by continually asking questions.

You have the power to choose your own destiny and the way you want to live your life. 2020 has been a year of introspection and the personal assessment of core values, quality of life decisions, and for many, the meaning of life itself. 2021 gives you the opportunity to take a stand for the life you want to live and what you are leaving behind as your legacy, and to do so; you must use this opportunity to seek information, stay informed, and get the answers you desire.

We will be confronted with many choices and decisions that will call upon our connection to our sovereign rights as people. Every voice matters, and everyone counts. My opinion is that leading from love and compassion does not mean acquiescence and fear of standing up. In fact, it may just mean the opposite. P.S. that is an opinion, not a fact.

THE UN-HABIT: TRUSTING EVERYTHING YOU HEAR OR READ

Why: Critical thinking is a skill that appears to be going out of fashion as many blindly follow what they hear or read without question.

One of the first criteria in true critical thinking is verifying the source of information. Many sources that we rely on are not neutral. Journalists, universities, media, etc., are all funded by interested parties. But, behind the funding and interests, there are ideologies, world views, and economic drivers that can skew the information. Ignoring rather than exposing the interlocking of directors, which is actually in contravention of anti-trust laws, is a case in point.

For example, the much-needed discussion on the efficacy, goals, and safety of vaccines is not covered by mainstream media channels. The SM moguls, who have interests in monitoring social behavior and opinions, have classified all discussion on the topic of vaccines as conspiracy theories and hereby censor open discussion in the name of protecting the public from misinformation.

Secondly, there is a difference between fact and opinion. The lockdowns were based on the Imperial College projection numbers and policy was not adjusted when the projections were wrong. The WHO changed the definition of Pandemic after the swine flu allowing governments to implement emergency orders. Naturopathic Doctors in Canada cannot talk about Covid-19 and immunity in the same sentence. These are all facts.

An opinion is what one believes about the facts they are presented with. For example, whether previously well-known and safe drugs, such as Ivermectin, which are being used clinically with positive results as a treatment for Covid should be stopped as they have not previously been tested for this particular use, is a matter of opinion.

Critical thinking allows us to ask why there is no funding for certain studies and why, despite numerous studies on the use of vitamin D, it is not being offered as the first line of defense. Facts are verifiable; opinions are debatable. In a censorship society, people follow narratives, opinions that have not withstood the test of debate or scientific scrutiny. Many opinions are not even allowed to be expressed.

Thirdly, information is being decontextualized. For example, cases in medical parlance is a word to denote symptomatic and affected individuals. "Cases" are not conventionally used to include a result of a test. The decontextualized use of increased "cases" leads to erroneous thinking.

Let's bring back critical thinking and weed out opinions from facts.

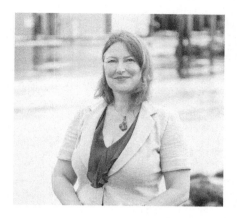

ABOUT MANON: While it is essential to verify our information, gain insight from actual life experiences, and what we witness, our most meaningful and important work is learning to connect to our senses. This starts by listening to our own bodies and becoming our own best second opinion. Now more than ever, we must embrace our innate healing ability and deep wisdom, which is the very essence of our beingness. While overcoming state 4 CA without pharmaceuticals or a hysterectomy, I discovered that we are accustomed to thinking that conflict resolution is mediated externally by experts. When it comes to health, it is an internal process.

10

PIVOT DAILY
CRISTIAN HAUSER

Why: The world has changed, and there is no turning back, but it also has brought people together more than before. We all faced the pandemic together, and we learned the value of essential workers and the value of having your loved ones near you.

But Covid has also brought a whole new generation of opportunities; as the world is changing, many businesses have learned to pivot into the new world.

With that, we also have to learn how to pivot our Habits. Good Habits are the foundation that builds your future. You can either have strong Habits that build you or face the consequences of your bad Habits.

One of the best Habits I learned from a covid world is complimenting someone and yourself. We have been sitting at home in our PJs, on zoom calls, and now many of us work from home. With that comes laziness. Laziness to even take care of ourselves and to appreciate who we are as people.

Many of us wake up every day, and the first thing we say when we look in the mirror is, "I look ugly, tired, etc." Not a great feeling, it makes us self conscious of who we are, and your confidence level goes out the window.

Now, what if, when you go to that same mirror and say, "Wow, who is that handsome/pretty face!" You will experience a whole new you. Your confidence level will be at an all-time high.

Most of the time, we praise celebrities, commenting on how they look "fabulous," but we forget the most important person, ourselves.

Words are power. What you say becomes real. If you keep telling yourself you are ugly or don't like what you see in the mirror, then your brain process it as a reality, and you will always go around believing you are less.

It works the same way if you tell yourself you are the very best and strong person. Your brain will manifest that you are a strong, beautiful person.

Imagine, if you use that same power of words and compliment someone else, you never know the impact you can have on someone if you just compliment them.

Daily I make a point to compliment someone. Many times people have stopped to tell me that the one compliment I gave them helped them through the day. You never know what someone is going through, and something as simple as a compliment can change their whole life.

When I built LiveGreatness, I had one goal in mind, to dress and inspire the people who will be changing the world. Our clothing is designed to inspire you every day to make you feel as though anything is possible.

Compliment yourself every morning, wear something that inspires you, and don't forget to compliment others.

We are all together in this, and the world will change, and you need to pivot to a new version of you, a more confident, powerful, and beautiful version of you.

This Habit is vital because the only thing better in the morning, other than a cup of coffee, is a good cup of confidence. Confidence helps us feel strong and encourages us to create a better version of ourselves. We thrive when we are feeling at our all-time high. Why not thrive every day?

Pivoting to a new world with new self-confidence is the power to get anything done and reach your goals.

Let's thrive at our all-time high, every day!

THE UN-HABIT: STOP THE EXCUSES

Why: No one really cares about the excuses you give about not moving forward. They only care about your actions. You can tell me that the reason you couldn't finish your month's goals was that you were too busy and didn't have enough time. In reality, all you are doing is making excuses because you did have the time, but instead, you spend it watching the next episode of your TV show or spend the whole day on social media looking for drama. You can make all the excuses in the world. In the end, you only are lying to yourself. Stop procrastinating and making excuses today, and your future self will thank you.

Imagine if you woke up tomorrow, and instead of making another excuse as to why you can't get up and do some exercises, you woke up and exercised for 5 to 10 minutes? I can guarantee you; it would be a life-changing experience when you make the first step into taking action.

Not only is taking action helping you build a stronger future, but it helps your current self-esteem realize that anything is possible if you stop the excuses and start working. Everyone has the same 24hrs of the day; there are not enough excuses you can give as to why you are not improving every day. Take 5 minutes every day and do one thing that will move you forward.

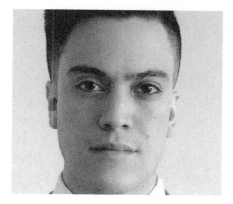

ABOUT CRISTIAN: By discovering the power of good mentorship and good Habits I've made over 1 million dollars in sales.

Cristian Hauser grew up in a small town in Peru with his grandfather, a fisherman, and although they didn't have much, he would always make it a Habit to get up early in the morning to make sure he could bring food to the table. He knew how important Habits are and how they can change who we decide to become.

11

THE POWER OF AFFIRMATIONS
ELIZABETH HARPER

Why: Every day, we affirm ourselves with our words whether we are aware of it or not. Your self-talk is heard and felt in your energy, which signals and attracts similar from the universe. What are you attracting with your words? What kind of health, people, circumstances, and events are you attracting with your words? Are you affirming failure without realizing it?

On average, 80% of our thoughts are habitual and negative, meaning that we repeat the same thoughts day in and day out well, without giving much thought to it! We get stuck in a habit loop of negative dialogue beginning when we wake up and continue through the day. Why?

Because our brains are wired to keep us safe, even if we are not in danger. For example, if you're thinking of joining a class, going to the gym, or perhaps writing a book, these are great intentions. Yet, your mind sees these constructive events as a threat because it's out of the ordinary. Strange but true.

You might find yourself affirming negatively charged expressions like "I am going to fail!" or "I feel foolish trying this." This usually happens when we want to do something out of our comfort zone.

And negative statements become habitual a lot faster than positive statements do. You see, our brains respond much quicker and powerfully to negative words because they threaten our survival and positive words do not. Even if we are doing something good for ourselves, our minds and bodies don't recognize our intentions, and the negative self-talk begins.

Don't get me wrong; we don't need to speak positively 24/7. There is a use for dissatisfaction, in fact, most of us have changed our lives for the better because we were dissatisfied with one thing or another, but we acted on what we wanted to change. Habitual negative self-talk leads to stuck emotions, sending out the wrong vibes, and shutting out what you do want.

Why is it important to make positive affirmations a daily habit? Because when we are in the habit of negative self-talk, we shut ourselves down and become stuck in our daily lives. We attract what we don't want, and we can make ourselves physically ill.

Positive affirmations are a fantastic initial practice towards a confident mindset and attracting the life you desire. When habitually practiced, positive affirmations physically re-wire the brain for expecting and attracting better.

How do we break this habit?

First, start with a small affirmation, then build consistency, then momentum. When forming a habit, pair it with a daily activity such as waking up, brushing your teeth, driving to work, going to bed, etc. This technique is called anchoring and is the best way to form a lasting habit.

For example, in the morning, when you first open your eyes, state your affirmation such as "I am attracting all that I need today." After a week or so, start saying your affirmation 3-5 times each and at various times in the day. Your affirmation doesn't have to be believable at first. Action works faster than changing your mindset. The belief will come later.

You are programming your mind to look and attract what you tell it to. Give your mind a command, and that's what it will keep looking for.

Have you ever tried to remember a song and then, days later, remembered it out of the blue? Even though you consciously forgot, you subconsciously gave your brain a command, and it kept looking for the answer. No matter where you are at or what you are doing, your mind will keep looking and working hard to give you an answer. So, if you habitually say things like "I am unlucky," your mind and the universe will prove you right.

So, here are some tips to make your habit even more powerful.

Pair affirmations with imagery, emotions, movements, and extra adjectives to engage the whole mind and body.

For example: State the affirmation "I am confident" right now. Now repeat it again but visualizing you acting confident, feeling optimistic, raising your hands in the air, and adding empowering adjectives; "I am confident, energized, and powerful!" Feel the difference?

So, as you go through your day, consider your negative self-talk; what affirmation can you add to be beneficial? What do I want to attract into my life?

Expectancy is a powerful magnet, and so are your words!

THE UN-HABIT: VISUALIZING FAILURE

Why: I'm going to begin by asking you to mentally see (visualize) a time you failed in something you genuinely wanted, and a time you felt you succeeded. Feel the emotions. Most likely, the first scenario felt bad, and you might have experienced negative physical sensations in your body, while the second scenario made you smile and feel lighter.

We tend to visualize future events going unfavorably. This primes our entire energy for failure, like a self-fulfilling prophecy. We become stuck, our heart rate rises, and we train our minds to expect disappointment. Now, I am no stranger to disappointment. I have experienced endless setbacks, disappointments, and obstacles, the likes that would make a very entertaining movie. I have, fortunately, observed many years ago my tendency to visualize the worse. And I am not alone in this habit. Especially during these unprecedented times, we can let our minds wander for the worse.

Visualization is a powerful tool: It can either prime us for success or stop us in our tracks. When we habitually visualize something potentially going wrong, our bodies and minds look for ways to adjust to do it and make it happen in the physical world. You don't want this!

The good news is, used properly, visualization raises confidence levels, so you're more likely to act. Even when we think we are limited, our minds will find a way to bust through limitations by visualizing being successful.

Studies have proven that people who visualize doing well instead of physically doing the same act have shown it can work just as well because your mind sees you making it repeatedly.

Many athletes make visualization a daily habit by practicing their sport in their minds and pushing past limitations. They create (and you can too) change in their mind before it happens. You can visualize and create a new life for yourself, so your mind will become familiar with it in real life.

So, how can we break this negative habit? Visualize differently!

Catch yourself when you're visualizing yourself failing and imagine being successful instead.

The more details you can add, the better. When visualizing, use strong emotions, smells, vivid colors, facial expressions such as smiling and movements such as clapping). Make this fun! This engages your whole mind and body.

If you find yourself visualizing bad things, give that part of yourself (negative mindset) a name like Fred or Carol and say,

"Now, Fred, you stop that!" Giving your negative mindset another name sets it apart from the real you. It'll make the negative habit easier to stop.

Successfully breaking a bad habit requires exchanging it for a good one. Begin exchanging (negatively visualizing) with (positively visualizing) so it will become familiar with you.

So, next time you find yourself imagining things going wrong, tell your Fred or Carol to stop and visualize yourself to success!

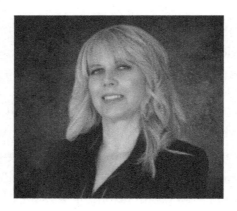

About Elizabeth: Elizabeth Harper is a confidence and manifesting coach, otherwise known as the "Confident Manifester." By combining confidence mindset and law of attraction practices, she offers a unique, powerful, and fun coaching platform for women who feel stuck in their lives.

Learning what confidence truly is and co-creating with the universe will transform you from a "self-doubter" to a "confident manifester." Let's take that vision in your mind and make it a reality!

12

BELIEVE IN YOU AND GO FOR IT!

JENNIFER JERALD

Why: It's the first massive step to making a giant pivot and changing your life.

Have you ever found yourself sitting in a daydream state? How about watching your favorite talent show, hearing your favorite song, or attending a dream event only to find yourself asking how you got there?

Do you feel like everyone else has it easier, and as much as you'd love to be able to do what they do, you can't, or you think you can't? Do you feel like everyone else has all the luck, and you're stuck at work at a job you don't love, but you do it because it's all you have and need to provide for your family?

Do you have dreams, and you know "if I only had the time," you'd be successful at it? Friends, this has been my life for almost 47 years. I have sat back, watched my dreams be played out by others, and complained about not having any luck and no time. For 15 years, I sat in my busy little nail salon in my home, just getting by. I loved my clients, I did excellent work but it wasn't enough.

Enter COVID, and everything changed on a dime. A statewide mandate shut down my salon and thousands of others. I was devastated and didn't know what to do. I had just published my first book, "Dare to H.E.A.L. Thriving with BPD" and immediately had to reflect back on its pages to "survive" the perceived blow to my future.

I thought of all the things I could do, wanted to do, and was trained to do. In a previous book, I talked about my success and being a director in the Tupperware business. I would rebuild. That would be the way for me to go. As I took the steps forward to be a leader in the company again, I realized this was NOT for me and NOT in alignment with my REAL DREAM. Almost as quickly as the world changed, I changed. I took the challenge of this change in momentum and realized I finally had the time I needed to believe in myself and go for it! I am a life long learner and now had extra time to consistently learn through additional courses, earned certifications, and grew through the change. I don't have to work for anyone else. I can be who I was meant to be. All I had to do was BELIEVE and GO FOR IT! Just believing isn't enough, but it's the first huge step to making a giant pivot and turning a disaster into destiny. The time is now. Believe it. Make the pivot. Stay consistent. Go for it! And watch your dreams become a reality.

THE UN-HABIT: GIVE IN TO DEFEAT

WHY: No success comes without some struggles.

In a song I wrote, "Sitting on the Sidelines," it says, "Perception is truth, what does yours say? Does it tell you that you're strong, or does it tell you that you're weak? Does it say that you're not perfect and there's no way to compete? Are you listening and accepting defeat? Are you sitting on the sidelines at war with yourself? Are your perceptions killing your dreams?"

In a pivotal moment and total career change, I cannot tell you how many times this portion of my song has run through my head the moment I gave in to defeat.

It is not always easy to see the gift in the garbage coming at you.

However, I can tell you that when you refuse to give in to defeat, you will not see obstacles. You will find strength and joy in the opportunities offered by occasional defeat. Defeat is not a permanent condition unless you succumb and stop believing in yourself. No amount of success comes without struggle. Nothing worth having comes without risk. No challenge in change comes without setbacks. The key to success is to keep moving, believing in you, and never, ever, ever giving into defeat.

The song continues, "No more sitting on the sidelines and missing your life, let your dreams take flight. Don't worry about perfection; mistakes are part of life! You have what it takes to go and live, live your life!" If we give in to defeat, we aren't living.

We are watching others live vicariously, and inadvertently our dreams go to an entity that isn't guarding them.

I'd like to share an excerpt from my book, "Dare to H.E.A.L.", as I talk about the feeling that others are luckier and more successful than I. It reads, "What I didn't realize is that there may have been some luck or they may have known some of the "right" people, but mostly it's because they didn't give up". They didn't let fear and naysayers shut them down. The world is full of miraculous stories of overcoming difficulties…and so much more! Friend…I want you to know, if I could look you in the eye today, I would tell you that YOU ARE ONE OF THEM! Your success story just hasn't been written yet!".

Are you ready to live your dreams? YES? Believe in you, let your dreams take flight and never give in to defeat!

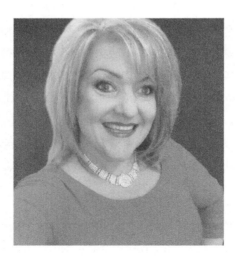

About Jennifer: Let's move you from living in fear to living the life of your dreams. Your transformation is waiting for you, to believe in you.

Life experience is one of the best teachers. Jennifer spent much of her life living in fear and has moved out of that state, now rising to help you do the same. Jennifer Jerald is known as the Fear to F.O.C.U.S. specialist who leads your way to a higher path.

"Although life can feel like a bareback bull ride, we can now take that bull by the horns, smack it on the fanny and say "giddy-up." The five-step Fear to F.O.C.U.S. program is your pathway to overcoming the challenges of your life by improving confidence, increasing success, and accelerating personal growth.

Jennifer Jerald is an international #1 Best-selling author, speaker, and dedicated transformational coach who knows what it takes.

13

PRACTICE INNER P.E.A.C.E.

AMBER YBARRA

Why: Practice Inner P.E.A.C.E. (Positive Mindset. Environment Awareness. Accountability. Clarity. EQ.) Inner peace starts with you. The acronym that best summarizes what has helped me and many others I've coached boils down to this practice when major stressors arise.

It's the idea of holding space for true P.E.A.C.E. that will enable you to go inward to move onward. With this, you can assess your life as it is now and then re-assess it with the intention to cultivate a life you're thriving in vs. a life you're merely trying to survive in.

The key here is to note where you feel you are with these 5 things now, then write out where you want to be and adjust accordingly. You can be in a completely different place in your lifestyle, health, love, happiness, spirituality, finances, career, and more if you first conquer these 5 things.

P.E.A.C.E. - Positive Mindset. Environment Awareness. Accountability. Clarity. Emotional Intelligence.

Each of these connected and applied will help you thrive during and post the global pandemic.

Positive Mindset: To have a positive mindset is the first step that will domino effect your life in a growth mindset direction. This does not mean toxic positivity or ignoring painful and uncomfortable situations. Rather, this means to shift your focus beyond any negative current circumstances, viewing the overall good in life, and then cultivating more of the good. Obtaining a positive mindset means you are intentionally choosing to approach your life, right now, with optimism for brighter days. Followed by action to create those brighter days with your mindset in a positive light.

Environment: Who and what you surround yourself with will create the well-being of your emotional and mental state of mind. Suppose the people you're constantly surrounded by are negative, depressed, and only talk about worst-case scenarios. In that case, that will ultimately paint the picture of your future. However, suppose you not only choose to be the light but surround yourself with friends, family, and an online community that lift you up. In that case, this will encourage you to see all the reasons why you too will thrive during this time.

Accountability: Taking ownership of your actions and letting other trusted peers hold you accountable will mean the difference between sinking or swimming. Having accountability enables you to be a leader in your life and to be resourceful enough to act on the change you want to see within it.

Clarity: Clarity is your direction. You cannot gain personal development without it, as it creates a path for your success. When you gain clarity, you are aligning your goals with your actions, thus making major headway to a fulfilled life, despite current circumstances.

Emotional Intelligence: Lastly, your emotional intelligence or EQ (emotional quotient) is the central link. If you cannot control your emotional state, you are not in control of your life. Acquiring EQ allows you to be around negativity such as the news, media, negative people, etc.... without becoming that. It allows you to observe but not be consumed by it. This allows you to hold enough space for your own emotions to process in self-awareness and self-regulated way.

THE UN-HABIT: CHANGE YOUR THOUGHTS AND TRAJECTORY

Why: The one most important thing you should un-Habit, are your reoccurring negative thoughts. According to the National Science Foundation, the average person has up to 60,000 thoughts per day. Of those thoughts, 95% are repetitive and negative thoughts.

Imagine what your day would look like if you changed the negative thoughts that cause you the same stressors, anxieties, and depressive feelings. If you even nipped one in the bud, this could change the course of your entire day, ultimate mood, and year.

Here are 5 ways you can do just that:

1.) *Stop negative thoughts in their tracks:* It's time to think of a solution and put your energy towards the change you want to see instead of dwelling on the worries you have carried from yesterday. To do this, take the next worry that pops into your mind, close your eyes, and imagine drawing a huge red X through that thought, then energetically toss it away. As you do this, choose to refocus on something good to clear out that negative thought to take its place.

2.) *Savor your small wins of the day:* You got out of bed at the time your alarm went off, got the mail, then also went through the mail, WIN. You waited on the phone for over 30 minutes to talk to a representative about that one bill you've been dreading to face, WIN. You have changed out of your pajamas and dressed up to attend the Zoom meeting more than half-dressed, WIN. Doing this will build your self-confidence and keep you motivated to win even grander milestones in your week.

3.) *Move your body for half an hour a day: This* is not about resolutions for your best body this year. Moving your body is a physiological kick start to enhancing your brain and mood, helping to release stress, depression, and anxiety for a higher feeling of your well-being. Thus, helping those negative thoughts fall by the wayside.

4.) *Connect with others:* You can stay connected while social distancing. In fact, you should be reaching out to others and finding a community of people to connect with now more than ever to keep from the negative effects of isolation. As mentioned in the 1Habit before this, being cognizant of the environment you've created for yourself, including the people you associate with, will determine the quality of your mental, emotional, and physical state of well-being. Connect with other like-minded people for the quickest way to brighten your mood and motivate your positive thoughts and connectedness.

5.) *Read & Write:* The truth is, reading books that interest you and are simultaneously giving you knowledge and motivation for your life. And life interests is one of the best ways to get your mind focusing on the right, more uplifting things. In the same way, reading can positively impact your thoughts. Writing out all your worries then replacing them with ways to uplift yourself and life, such as writing positive affirmations and gratitude. Doing these will not only replace your negative with positive thoughts but reset your mood entirely for a better day entirely.

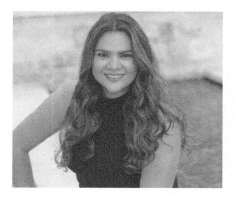

About Amber: Amber Ybarra is the American author of "Thriving into Thirty" and Podcast Host of The Positive Platform.

Through her brand and The Positive Platform, Amber helps other female entrepreneurs reinvent themselves through high-performance strategies and confidence building to scale their business.

Amber has spoken on stages and in communities throughout the world on this very topic. She continues to work with TEDx organizations and hosts physical and online events while teaming up with other trailblazing female leaders to share this growth process.

If you are a female entrepreneur tired of being scared to show up for your biggest goals and need help building a business strategy and gaining confidence to scale, Amber would love to book a discovery call with you today.

14

PLANT NEW SEEDS EVERY DAY
MARIE F. CELESTIN

Why: Can you imagine what you can harvest when you plant new seeds every day? At the start of the pandemic, I was stressed out and overwhelmed by a heightened level of uncertainty that I never experienced before.

I was homeschooling for the first time and was looking for a fun way to keep my kiddo engaged. More importantly, I wanted us to play and learn together as we figure out how to cope. We created a ritual of planting new seeds every day to give us a reason to go outside and design a little oasis while in isolation.

Every time I plant a seed, I feel more connected to my inner self, my son, and the outside world. This Habit is important because it gives me something fresh to look forward to daily. It amplifies my sense of wonder and curiosity in nature. As we spend more time outdoors together, we became more excited about the birds and butterflies we were attracting in our flourishing garden. They were, in fact, the only welcoming visitors without a mask.

Day by day, we witness our seeds poking their heads through the soil to eventually blooming into flowers and veggies. Besides the pure joy that it brought us to watch what we plant grow, this Habit's best benefit is feeling less stressed and becoming more mindful about what we focus our energy on.

This practice transforms how I start my day, how I bond with my son, become more open to connecting with new people, and inspired a renewed optimism about life. In essence, planting new seeds helps me discover sacred self-care and what truly matters regardless of the chaos in the world.

As long as I keep planting seeds, a promising future is possible. You, too, have the power to transform through this powerful Habit.

THE UN-HABIT: GET OUT OF YOUR COMFORT ZONE TO GROW

Why: You can't afford to keep this Habit if you have big dreams.

Are you willing to do what it takes to get out of your comfort zone? It's time to let it go NOW to make room for your gifts. It's such a game-changer when you acknowledge an old habit that no longer serves you and intentionally decide to pivot in the pursuit of the best version of you. You can still do it while scared and shaking.

This move has to be a conscious choice that demands consistent action to break it for good. I know change is hard, but you know what's worse, being stuck in the same place wishing for better year after year.

I remember eleven years ago, I was a new mom who just got laid off from my first job in healthcare and didn't know how I was going to feed my son. My whole world felt apart within minutes of getting that pink slip. I wasn't prepared for this level of impact while juggling family life and stress. I was comfortable in a safe job with benefits and never prepared for impact.

Fortunately, there was no time to have a pity party and feel sorry for me. I had to quickly get out of my comfort zone and try a new line of work to make ends meet. Scared or not. Ready or not. My number 1 priority was to take care of my son, no matter what.

When you get hit with a curveball like that, you don't have the luxury to dwell, blame other people or get stuck in coulda, shoulda, and woulda. It is done! It was time to pull up my big girl's pants and figure it out. Even in crisis, you have a choice on how you respond, plant a seed, and stay in action. Sometimes we make the boldest, most courageous badass decision when life throws us a curveball. I had to get out of my comfort zone real quick because feeding my kid put me in do or die goddess mode.

This Habit of getting out of your comfort zone will build your resilience muscles and fuel a fire in your belly to be MORE than your struggles. There's no going back once you tap into your strengths and remain open to new possibilities. Once you release this old Habit, you will soar in momentum.

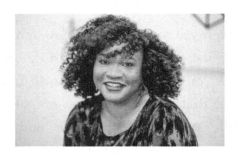

About Marie: Marie Celestin, affectionately known as the "Goddess of Self-care", is a wellness coach and creator of Talk! with Marie Podcast. As a result of her coaching, stressed-out clients go from burnout and brain fog to mindfulness, emotional eating to improving their gut health and prioritizing sacred self-care while flourishing in momentum. I'm looking for people who are ready to release stress from their life and rediscover what brings them joy. Who do you know?

15

IF IT'S TO BE, IT'S UP TO ME

LYNN MARYSH

Why: Say "If it's to be, it's up to me" when you have aspirations for success but don't feel like doing something you should do.

Things happen in life that will bring your down. Sometimes unexpectedly. You are totally responsible for the success of your life. There are no excuses. There may be set backs or problems that come up, but dealing with them as they happen, in a 'calm and centered' manner, will have you build the confidence you need to develop new skills and habits in resolving such problems, should they come up again.

Family dynamics change, as do friends and jobs - keep your thinking in the moment and your focus on your goal, and in so doing, you will weather out any 'storm'.

While some things will definitely have an impact on you, it's important to realize that some things are beyond your control.

It's up to you, and you alone, to accept responsibility for the success of your life, and this will come from the way you deal with things. No matter how bad you might have it, no matter what difficulties or challenges you might encounter, there are many people who have had difficulties and challenges far greater than you are ever likely to encounter, and somehow, they manage to pull through. And you can do the same.

Remember... "If it's to be, it's up to me."

That simple one-line sentence says it all. It places the responsibility exactly where it should be... directly on your shoulders.

Make a total commitment to your success. Once you have made the decision to be successful, be successful.

Do it with both feet in. Don't let anything hold you back.

Even more than being successful, see that success gets in you. Make a commitment that you are going to succeed, no matter what.

Don't try to work different methods at one time; choose a path, and stick to it. You can't do justice to more than one at a time, and if you try to, you'll likely end up frustrated and never know whether you could have been successful.

THE UN-HABIT: SAYING I'M NOT GOOD ENOUGH

Why: Your programming is most likely as a result of some well intended individual but now you have to see that you are good enough. There are no excuses. You are not them, and they are not you.

Take control of your time. Time is an expendable commodity. Each one of us has the same 24 hours each day. When those hours are gone, they cannot be replaced. They are gone forever, never to be recaptured.

You must treat your time as precious and guard it wisely and selfishly. Don't let anyone disrupt you or take you away from the focus you have on the success of your life.

People who don't have goals are used by people who do. If you let others draw you away from your goals, you are saying that their goals are more important than your own. And That is enough to cause you to live a life of mediocrity and make you miserable. Communicate in a loving manner to people demanding of your time that you desire and need to focus on what it is you plan to achieve and the time you require to achieve it. This may be a little more challenging if you are trading time for money when working for someone else, but during your off time when developing yourself to be independent, plan your work and work your plan.

If you are serious about your success – really serious, then Time is one of the most important and critical areas to defend.

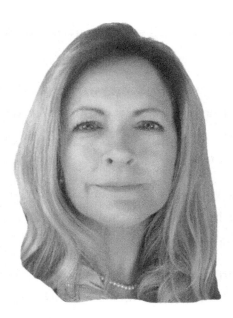

ABOUT LYNN: Lynn Marysh will have you shift your perspective from one of breakdown to one of breakthrough for most conversations when someone is feeling stuck.

16

FOLLOW YOUR DREAMS
CHRISTINA KUMAR

Why: Follow your dreams because you're the only one who can do it. I was expected to become a doctor or lawyer, but that is not the path I wanted to pursue for myself. I had to push for what I wanted, even though it was not what others had planned for me. Deep inside, I knew I wanted something else. I knew I wanted to go on a different path. So, on the journey, I began. My ultimate goal of being an entrepreneur and entertainer started out slowly and with many twists. I wasn't handed anything and had to earn everything, but it was worth it because I had many dreams come true. I had once competed in a 54-hour entrepreneur's competition powered by Google with total strangers; this was one of the best things I had done at the time. It had totally shattered the shell I had. I had to speak publicly, resolve conflicts, and create a company all in 54 hours! Want to know how I did it? By remembering to follow my dreams! The strong desire to follow my dreams made me push past my doubts because I wanted to make sure that I had given my dreams a fighting chance. I won 1st place and learned so many things that I can use to this day. Most importantly, it gave me the confidence I needed and lifelong friendships.

Following your dreams is a life-long journey, and your dreams can change. What you once wanted as a child can be totally different from what you want today, and that is completely okay! If I got what I wanted as a child, I would have many headaches right now. Luckily, I now know my most important goals and will ultimately benefit not only myself but also others.

THE UN-HABIT: STUBBORN MINDSET

Why: As I write this on New Year's Eve, I remember how much of a change 2020 brought both good and bad. I went through the many positive life changes that have occurred this year and am grateful for all the good that has occurred. The saying "bend and not break" has never been so true. Most of us have learned this year to be more flexible and patient and look out for others. This year we realized the need and importance of a healthy community. We also realized the need to take care of ourselves and the planet. This is a positive change we should take into 2021.

Change, however, cannot occur with a stubborn mindset. This pandemic has taught us that we need to be flexible and more open to other ways of doing things if they are ethically sound.

Having a stubborn mindset can bring undue stress and block helpful solutions to problems. When we let go of having a stubborn mindset, not only can we relax more; we can breathe. Sometimes changes are difficult, but they can be a solution to problems. We all want change to be easy and pleasant, but many times that is not the way change happens. Many people will wait until it is too late to change; you want to make sure that does not happen.

Life is a journey with many twists and turns. We want to make sure we make the right decisions and become everything we want to be. Being rigid as well as stubborn will most likely lead to difficulties and hurt relationships. Practicing being flexible and learning to change a stubborn mindset can help in more ways than one and create stronger relationships. If you can minimize having a stubborn mindset and learn to "bend and not break," you can also help create a better you!

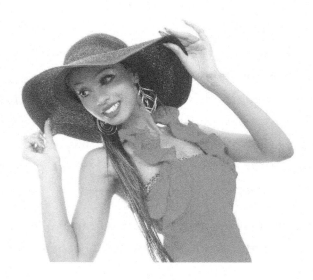

ABOUT CHRISTINA: Christina Kumar is the owner of Christina Kumar PR where she helps those who want to expand their business and reach. Christina Kumar PR has experience helping Olympic athletes, CEOs of international companies, and award-winning musicians among others to land media attention that they need to expand their products, projects, and services. Email: info@christinakumar.com for more information.

17

AUDIBLY GIVE THANKS FOR AWAKENING AND YOUR SENSES

DR DEB CARLIN

Why: When you practice authentic gratitude, it shifts your brain activity with an increase in the experience of mental discipline which leads to greater happiness as you realize the control you have to direct your thoughts. Gratitude that is authentic is that which you speak in sincerity, there is no resistance to your thoughts, your words, and the feelings associated with them that come from your heart. They are indeed the only thing in life that you have absolute control over.

Yes indeed this is a type of mind game because you need to understand that your thoughts become you. Your mind and your heart must be in harmony for genuine, anything, about you to exist. Adopt the belief that your heart emits an energy and your mind processes it, allow the good feelings to flow.

Once you develop this habit, it generalizes into other aspects of your mind body health as you feel inspired and then motivated to engage further the actions that promote wellness, joyfulness, and optimism. There is a beautiful contagion which occurs – within you!

Interestingly, the intrinsic rewards that you discover continue to give rise to new creative ways to feel better, explore more appreciation and attract people and projects into your life because you exude a good vibe. In quantum physics, this is measurable as a high frequency.

The most beautiful aspect of this habit is that it is grounded in mind body science which has revealed that our endocrine, neurological, cardiovascular, respiratory, digestive, integumentary, immune, muscular, renal, reproductive, and skeletal systems all respond to our thoughts and feelings. We promote that which we think and feel – comfort or disease.

Attitude is everything and you're shifting into a good one is easy -- just start right now. Snap your fingers, shake your head, proclaim out loud – I am good, I am love, I am enough. Own it in peace and with a smile that extends from the inside out.

THE UN-HABIT: STOP THE NEGATIVE THOUGHTS AND STATEMENTS!

Why: The most essential component of this habit is that it is so powerful because indeed -- you hear what you say -- every single word of it. And as you hear it, your mind believes it and stores it and rehearses whatever you said. The influence of the mind over the body is astonishing and tangible.

Sit here for a moment as you read these words and recall the times in your life when you have made yourself sick with worry, angst, anger, and negativity. You have given yourself headaches, acid indigestion, stomach aches, constipation, heart pains...and what else? These are not the experiences that you have during times of genuine peace and comfort and happiness.

We each need to be aware and consistently careful. You cannot afford the luxury of a negative thought. Not ever.

When you are negative in any manner, you are firing negative neurons in your brain and giving them strength. You are lowering your energetic frequency, which is measurable, and as you do so you become susceptible to the list of illnesses mentioned and when prolonged, that list intensifies.

As your negativity increases, the level of acidity in your body increases because you are eliciting the stress response and releasing chemical reactions based on what your body thinks is real even though the threats are only taking place inside of your mind. The experience of negativity proceeds into worry, anxiety, anger, despair, and lands in a state of depression if left to travel that far. It is a short road to arrive at and a long journey to return from and land back in happiness.

Stop. Stop every negative thought and every negative speak -- snap your fingers as swiftly as you start to go negative and immediately turn it 180 degrees to the positive.

It is easy -- just do it!

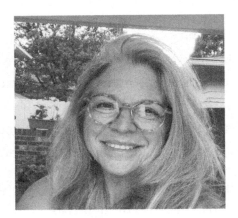

About Deb: Dr Deb Carlin authored Build the Strength Within, a program designed to introduce you to the very core of how awesome you are. With an actual Blueprint that emulates one you would have created to build your home, this one has you building you, your health and the life you dream about.

Alongside the book, there are videos and audio files. Most importantly and enjoyably, there is a highly engaging online course where you feel very attended to and guided into your success.

18

I AM DOING A GREAT JOB
DR. FRANCESCA RICHARDSON

Why: You are at home interacting with you. Whatever you are facing, a difficult project a tedious day on zoom, a critical boss... Say to yourself, "I am doing a great job!" You can picture those who care about you saying this to you too, and smiling at you.

Why? The short answer is, this encourages you and we all need encouragement.

But I am going to give you a longer answer with a personal story, and research! About 10 years ago, I had the crazy thought that I wanted to go get a PhD to do research to help people. But it was expensive, and the math and statistics it entailed had always stopped me. In addition, I have long been a 'C' or 'D' student at math, but I never really understood why. I always had questions my teachers could not understand like "which side of the 1 should I start on to count to get the next number?"

or "if the zero doesn't exist, how do I count it?" I probably would have done better counting something tangible, like blocks, (and that is a story for another day) but it shows why I struggled. So with a great tutor, and a goal in mind, I told myself "You are doing a great job!" and I aced that GRE test and got a full scholarship for my PhD!

But since I am a researcher, as well as a psychotherapist and coach, I don't expect you to take my word for it, I have to look up the research so I can prove it to you and to me! Turns out there is a lot of research on how encouragement of others helps the person being encouraged. In the research, this idea is called 'self-encouragement' or encouragement of the other person's self. One research article stated "self-encouragement is a strong predictor of hope and mental health and can help better resist against the physical and psychological crises." Research has shown it increases creativity in employees, helps mothers cope with illness in their sick children, relieves depression in psychiatric inpatients, and helps patients in stroke recovery. Wow, if it can help in these varied and severe situations, do you think it will help in your home office with mood, motivation and productivity?

I hope the answer is Yes! But okay, you are alone in your home office, there is only you! So what about encouraging yourself? Turns out research would put this under 'self-compassion,' which makes sense, as compassion covers all sorts of positive empathic feelings and approaches -- to others as well as oneself -- of which encouragement would merely be one expression. Yes, research shows self-compassion provides positive outcomes. So have a little self-compassion – and self-encouragement -- or a lot --and express it through encouraging yourself!

You can be the champion of you! Un-habit the negative self-talk, as this merely makes you feel bad about yourself and unmotivated. Start the new Habit of positive self-talk!

The Un-Habit: Negative self-talk

Why: Many people want to leave a 'legacy.' What legacy do you want to leave? One legacy has to do with how you treat others. People remember how you made them feel. Do you help others feel good about themselves in interaction with you? If you help yourself feel good, if you are talking positively to yourself, if you are happy and healthy, then you can treat other people well.

But negative self-talk can be a hard habit to break without deeper understanding. Many times, negative self-talk develops from how we were treated early in our lives. Sometimes we were influenced by how we saw others being treated. Oddly enough, if we were bullied, criticized, abused, humiliated -- even by people who seemed to care about us -- we may have begun to give ourselves the same negative treatment. This is learned behavior, and we repeat it as a kind of defense. Amazingly, we can begin to act like those bullies because they seemed to have power. Also, sometimes the people who bullied or criticized us were people we loved, but they may have been bullied themselves as children. Or they may have been in the midst of an addiction, mental illness, poverty, or have had some other problem that made it hard for them to be kind to themselves and others. In addition, if they were our family members – we may have emulated them or wanted to make them 'right.' This is childhood logic, and we are not conscious of it when we are adults. However, the belief that may develop as a child is that if we bullied ourselves inside our minds, then we were more likely to act small, and be less likely to be bullied by those around us. But this not work well when we become adults we need to be assertive and treat ourselves and others well.

So stop the bullying! Start with yourself. Your positive words to others will hold more value if you feel confident and at peace because you are talking with love and care to yourself inside. When you develop the self-discipline of positive self-talk, you help yourself feel better, and you can show and teach self-love. Bring that self-love to every interaction, and the legacy you leave is that you can teach others to love themselves.

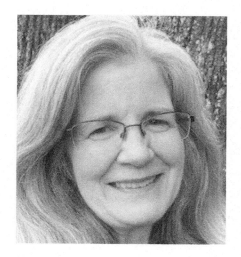

ABOUT FRANCESCA: I'm known as the Therapist's Therapist and Dream Activator. Because – as a psychoanalyst, hypnotherapist, and researcher, and for over 30 years, I have helped people to heal issues stored deep within them. One major way I work is to help you overcome your INNER CRITIC ---(which has resulted in a lack of confidence) --- to achieve peace, emotional freedom, and personal success. I teach people to kick out the negative self-talk and embrace 'yes' to their inner champion.

19

FAIL FORWARD WITH RELENTLESS ACTION.

SHERRI LEOPOLD

Why: Failing Forward requires relentless action. Success demands imperfect action 99% of the time. Creating success requires trial and error. In fact, failures are the training ground for high-level success. Charles Kettering stated, "An inventor fails 999 times, and if he succeeds once, he's in. He treats his failures simply as practice shots." Look at Thomas Edison. He 'failed' 10,000 before he was able to make the incandescent lightbulb work correctly, something we today take completely for granted! He said the previous attempts were all just unsuccessful experiments. He failed forward with every single attempt. This is the very definition of imperfect action. He continued to act not because it always worked, but because his goal never changed, and he BELIEVED he could make it happen. Post-Covid, so many things have changed. Have your goals changed? Ultimately, it doesn't matter if they have; what can't change is your commitment to fail forward with relentless action. Will you have to adjust 100 times? Will you have to try 10,000 times to get something right? You might just have to do that! If you want to accomplish, create, or invent something, you don't change your desire to do it simply because it doesn't work the first few times. Realistically, it might require MORE attempts post covid than any other time in history. The landscape of our lives is very fluid right now and changing daily. We must change with it and go with the flow, be in flow if you will, to persevere through difficulty and failure. Fail forward with consistent daily action. This means, even if it feels like it isn't working, do it anyway. If it feels hard, do it anyway. Many times, we don't KNOW what we don't know until we learn we didn't know it. That is precisely why failing forward and continuing to attempt to win every day with relentless action is the key to living in a post covid world. You will never find your way by standing still and doing nothing. I say this often, "Do nothing, get nothing. Do something, and you will get something. Even if it it's not what you wanted, you will have something to work with."

THE UN-HABIT: QUIT STARTING AND STOPPING!

Why: Post covid- our culture doesn't tolerate starting and stopping anymore. Patience for such a thing is long gone. The very reason Thomas Edison was eventually successful with the light bulb is that he never quit. He didn't start and stop; he simply revised it and tried again. If you want to write a book, you will struggle if you write every day for a week and then do not pick it up for a month. Momentum is born of continuous efforts strung together. Because the world is in such a fluid state, if you stop and try to start later, what might have worked then may not work now. Starting and stopping kills momentum, but it also kills enthusiasm. You need to have joy in your journey. Joy is not found with starting and stopping. The gaps merely provide space for frustration, regret, and doubt to set in and reside. Starting and stopping is a killer in most businesses and in relationships. Relationships, like businesses, need consistent attention, time, and effort. They do not fare well on a sometimes basis. Especially with Covid, people have become acutely aware of what is available to them through the internet. If they don't like your service, they will go find ten other people happy to serve them. If your customers don't feel they are worthy of consistent attention, they will go elsewhere. If you are in a relationship and you don't give it time and attention, the relationship will wither. Relationships do not survive starting and stopping, they also require relentless action.

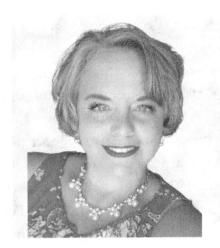

ABOUT SHERRI: My name is Sherri Leopold; I am the leader of the Stop Self Bullying Movement, 200K Leader with Le-Vel, and the host of Outside the Box with Sherri, where I shine a light on others making a difference in the world. It has always been my mission to serve others. I proudly help busy entrepreneurs plug in their own power cord. I help people Stand UP and Stand Out in their lives mentally, physically, and financially. Through public speaking and personal and group mentorship, I help uncover their limiting behaviors and help them S.N.A.P. out of the patterns that don't serve them. Are you living the life you deserve?

20

LOOK FOR THE SOLUTION

JACQUELIN BUCKLEY

Why: Serving time in the military taught me many different mindset strengths. For example, how to be dependable, reliable, and accountable. Now while my childhood taught me the critical mindset to be a problem solver, the military reinforced that ability for me. Problem-solving has become an innate Habit that I am incredibly grateful for. In my current profession as a mental health practitioner, I often see clients who come in with various problems and often cannot see beyond it. Interestingly, the solution to the problem appears very clear to all around them. However, they focus on the issue and not a possible solution that clouds the ability to see the answers they hold.

While it may seem odd that this occurs, it is quite common and normal. Because when we are in a state of chaos and our emotions have taken over; we cannot access the rational problem seeking part of our brain. Our thoughts continue to focus on the issue, making everything else continue to spiral out of control. With the pandemic, those who have been solution focused have continued to navigate the inconveniences because they have found alternate solutions. Those who have been laser-focused on the problem have allowed the inconveniences' to control their abilities ultimately. Finding a solution will enable us to take pride in knowing that we can think outside the box. It allows us to be happy, knowing that we can still be satisfied while we are uncomfortable. Seek to find solutions and celebrate the victory rather than focusing on the problem and becoming the victim.

When you can look at solutions and problem solve, you remove your ability to call yourself a victim to a challenge or problem. By taking the time to analyze and seek out alternate solutions, you empower yourself to survive and thrive during challenging times. When we can handle situations and find alternate solutions, we recognize that even some of the things we thought were enormous challenges are mere obstacles. Those obstacles are often placed in our path to either teach us something significant about ourselves or share the solution with others going through the same challenge.

THE UN-HABIT: STOP NUMBING UNCOMFORTABLE

Why: How do you deal with stress, anxiety or even having a crappy day? Do you go home and drink a bottle of wine and pass it off as "I deserve it, I worked hard"? Perhaps you buy things online, and the Amazon driver no longer needs his navigation system to get to your home. Or maybe you spend hours and hours watching TV or scrolling on social media. Or perhaps you find yourself snacking all day long on foods that give you moments of joy only to feel guilty later. For many years before finally being diagnosed with PTSD caused by my military mission participation, I found myself numbing my emotions. I shopped to gain moments of feeling happy and spent time out with friends more than being at home with my family. I could do anything to make the emotional turmoil I was feeling; go away for even a brief moment. I had to look healthy and like I had it all together, only breaking apart inside.

The problem with emotional numbing is that the sadness, guilt, shame, or other emotions we are feeling still stay with us even if we try and replace it with some of the unhealthy coping mechanisms I shared above. Those difficult emotions don't go away just because we pretend they don't exist. They will still be there after the shopping trip, the glasses of wine, when our social media connections are busy or after binge-watching Netflix. During this pandemic, I have observed that many individuals are numbing their emotions because they find what is happening very difficult to grasp or manage. They are being faced with many difficult situations and perhaps feel overwhelmed. They show they are thriving on the outside yet hiding on the inside by numbing the emotional pain they may be feeling. I would encourage you to practice connecting with your emotions and making it a daily habit to recognize your feelings. Journal about it, be brave, and talk about it but don't numb it with things that will be unhealthy in the long term. When you become aware and are able to acknowledge that you are not feeling at your best, you allow yourself to connect with yourself on an emotional level. Creating healthy habits will generate healthier results than emotional numbing with things that give us short term happiness.

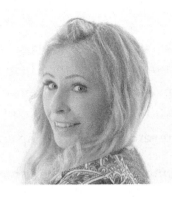

About Jacquelin: Jacquelin is a Motivational Speaker, Mental Health Professional and Resiliency Coach who; through the power of her story, inspires and shares successful tips to first responders for preventing & overcoming burnout and operational stress injuries while building resilience.

Jacquelin Buckley, CD, B.A., M.A. Counselling Psych, CCC is a Veteran, Best Selling Author, Mental Health Professional and Solopreneur who personally understands how burnout and stress can directly impact family, self and the ability to communicate effectively with others. As a volunteer with the Memory Project, Jacquelin has had several opportunities to speak at various events sharing her story on how she overcame Post Traumatic Stress Disorder's darkness. She emphasizes encouraging others who may be struggling with other various Operational Stress Injuries.

21

TAKE THE OPPORTUNITIES YOU HAVE
NICOLE BACZKOWSKA-POPELKA

Why: Every day, we face plenty of opportunities; many of them are good for us and might even change our lives. But a lot of the time, fear, or being busy, or being tired holds us back from taking those opportunities that are being dropped in our lap. It is essential to take these opportunities because they can change your life for the better.

I reluctantly went to model in my first fashion show. The night before, I acted like I was going to the gallows and not a fashion show. I felt that I was smart, and in college, what use would modeling be to me. I was so wrong. That one fashion show led me to do others, and I have had the opportunity to meet amazing people and have countless once in a lifetime experiences. I hate to say it but my mom signing me up and dragging me to that show was one of the best things she could have done for me. It makes me think how many more opportunities have I missed because I was tired, comfortable, or fake busy. How many fantastic opportunities are passing us by simply because we don't take them?

More often, people regret not doing something in comparison to doing something. Living life with regrets that you didn't take the chance is not worth it. Especially when those opportunities you are letting pass by can make your life so much more thrilling and lively. No one wants to live a boring life, and yet, many people settle into a monotonous cycle of comfort and familiarity, not willing to change what they are doing even if they are unhappy with their life.

When someone hands you an opportunity, don't take it lightly because it won't be there forever. If someone is giving you an opportunity, it means they see something in you that you probably don't see in yourself. It's time to jump on that opportunity that could change your life forever. What do you have to lose?

THE UN-HABIT: STOP BEING ASHAMED OF WHO YOU ARE

Why: Apparently, I eat cereal wrong. This is how I eat cereal to this day: I don't eat the colored or very sugary cereals, I warm up the milk on the stove, and I pour the milk into the bowl before the cereal, which is exactly the opposite of how the average American eats their cereal. I learned this valuable life lesson in 6th grade at a friend's sleepover birthday party. It was a normal middle school sleepover; we didn't really sleep, ate way too much junk food, and played truth or dare, which got ridiculously out of hand (someone almost threw up because they drank a concoction of all the condiments out of the fridge) everything was fine until breakfast. Breakfast was cereal, and it should have been ridiculously easy. However, I wasn't allowed to eat colored cereals as a kid. But here I was at a table teeming with sugar and red food dye, and to top it off, was a huge gallon of milk on the table. This was a scene I had never seen before in my life, and I had no idea what to do. So I asked the mom if she could warm up the milk for me, she looked at me like I had asked her for a unicorn, and I spent the rest of the morning being mocked by my peers that I ate cereal wrong. It's a silly story to bring up, but it is an experience that is tattooed into my brain. It was one of the many experiences that reminded me that I was different and did not fit in. Unfortunately, instead of being okay with it, I was ashamed of it. I felt that there must be something wrong with me if I couldn't even eat cereal like a "normal" person.

When people are ashamed, they paralyze themselves from going forward. There are some times where I still go back to the eating cereal experience and hold myself back from doing something in a way that makes sense to me. When you're ashamed of who you are, you spend your energy hiding who you are from the world instead of focusing your energy on growing yourself and making the world a better place. This is a great loss because the world desperately needs you in it. The world desperately needs people who want to make the world a better place, people who want to grow, and people who want to see the beauty in this world. The moment people are ashamed of who they are, the whole world misses out on how fantastic you are. Even worse, you sabotage your chance at being able to make a difference in your life or someone else's. In short, the world needs people that are willing to eat their cereal the wrong way and be empowered by it.

So many people are so much stronger, more powerful, more beautiful, and have significantly more life in them than they allow themselves to live. If you stop being ashamed of who you are, you'll finally be able to be free in your own skin. Finally, be able to pursue your dreams and passions without shame holding you back. Finally, be able to look in the mirror and love who you see. Finally, be able to help the people you want to help or live the way you want to live.

Imagine having the freedom to dream so big that you can inspire others to do the same, all because your own shame does not hold you back. What would your life look like? What kind of world would we live in if everyone stopped being ashamed of what made them different from everyone else? That's the life we should lead and the world we should want to live in—a life where we were empowered by our differences instead of being divided by them.

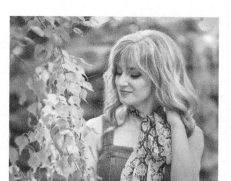

ABOUT NICOLE: My name is Nicole Popelka, and I'm known as the specialist of simplifying your home. My expertise is decluttering, reorganizing, redesigning, and redecorating your home. Allow me to be a part of your journey of reinventing your home, so you have more time and space to create more wonderful memories.

22

SEEK WISE, SPIRITUAL COUNSEL

MELISSA "THE MOTIVATOR" MACKEY

Why: Life is short.

You ever had that moment where you dropped to your knees, begging and pleading for things to be different, wishing you had wise counsel to help you listen, seek and find the answers? Your current situation does not need to define your destiny. The pandemic has proved to be challenging in many ways, but there's a blessing amidst the chaos. Are your eyes ready to see through a different lens? Are your ears prepared to hear potent, new, encouraging messages, and would you seek the wise counsel your soul is craving?

For many moments in my life, I thought it was over.

I drowned myself in debt, despair, and hopelessness, wondering how I'd ever make it through. My body succumbed to alcohol to the point of blackout, and I ingested drugs to numb it all out. My wild child, promiscuous life led me to feel emotionally bankrupt, physically exhausted, and spiritually dead. Too often, I was on my knees, begging and pleading for things to be different. I was tired of doing it all alone. I had to seek wise, spiritual guidance that would nourish me through my troubling times. The people I was currently associating with were stuck in the same darkness. My heart was empty, and I had no vitality pumping through it.

Most humans desire to reach the destination of peace, love, and joy while experiencing success. I believe it is through much grace and wise counsel that each of us will powerfully thrive post-pandemic. Grace does not come without having a faith that carries us through a crisis. Grace and wise counsel give us the supernatural strength to pivot.

Ask yourself WHO can I surround myself with daily to empower, uplift & support me?

You are the sum of the 5 closest people in your life.

Are you flooding your mind with news, media, and people that constantly complain and wonder why you feel drained?

For me, I seek spiritual mamas who are anchored and grounded in God and seek HIS wise wisdom daily. These mamas have been the lifeline that saved my soul, renewed my mind, and rewired my hurting heart. They impart strength into me when I feel weak and light my way during the dark times. My earthly, spiritual mamas have helped me listen with new ears, seek the right wisdom and counsel, and find a direct connection to the heavenly realm.

When you ignite your spirit with wise counsel, they have the ability to spark love, joy, and peace inside of you, post-pandemic. They teach you that when your heart fills with joy, your overflow of love pours into ALL areas of your life, creating abundance. Seek your counsel daily.

Align with the right people and, most importantly, give yourself grace so that you can rest in the place to hear the answers you're looking for. My Faith has been my healer, and post-pandemic, your spirit yearns for more. Tap in. Tune out. Turn on.

The Un-Habit: Stop the blame, shame & complain train

Why: Shaming is running rampant. Complaining seems to be the name of the game, and blaming is close behind. This pandemic has created a ripple through humanity that is constantly looking for what's not working, who to blame, and then feeling ashamed. Your job is to rise above the blame, shame & complain train.

The only way to peace, love, and joy is to seek the blessing. Find the gift inside the pandemic. You haven't had to jump on a plane for another event, engagement, or teaching. You've prayed for more family time; you got it. You wanted to be home more; you were blessed with the lockdown. You wanted to connect more to your spiritual self; the time was given.

It's time to tune in, pay attention to your own self-talk, and course-correct when you find yourself about to blame or complain. If your heart is set on blaming, shaming, and complaining, there is no room for you to receive abundance, opportunity, or blessings. The name of the game is love. Love moves mountains. It changes hearts. It's unconditional. When you operate from a place of love, you meet others where they're at. You're not shaming; You're honoring. You're not blaming; You're embracing. You're not complaining; you're giving thanks.

Those who focus on gifts are given more. You raise the vibration for the atmosphere you desire to create. Others are attracted to this. You have the power within to change your reality. The simple shift from blame, shame & complain to thanks and gratitude has the power to transform all time and space. Meet others where they are, come from a place of love, and witness miracles unfold post-pandemic.

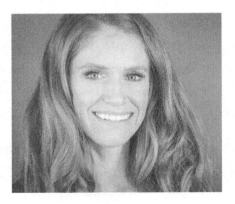

About Melissa: Melissa Mackey is a single mama on a mission to blaze a trail and empower women to tap into their God-given talents. Melissa helps plan, produce, and promote offline and online events, masterminds, and retreats. With close to 500 events under her belt, she is committed to teaching women how to make money through travel, marketing & media. She understands the power of building strong communities, meaningful relationships, and friendships that last a lifetime.

23

CONNECT WITH FIVE PEOPLE DAILY

BRENDA MARIE SHELDRAKE

Why: Covid made us all a bit more independent and isolated. That slight hint of fear that passes through the heart when somebody sneezes or coughs a bit too deeply. Those fears validated the messages we heard to stay in our homes and keep to ourselves – to stay safe! We isolated – locking the doors, only leaving the house to pick up the necessities. We thought we were staying safe, but that safety comes at a high price!

Humans aren't meant to spend their days alone. Mothers with small children, the elderly, and those with no family came to see this safety as a prison sentence. Reruns on the television and the endless broadcast of Covid numbers, predictions of the doom as death numbers climbed brought us all to a place of fear and a creeping lack of hope.

Would the life we knew ever return? How were we going to stimulate our brains? Worst of all, that sense of connection, the joy of helping another human, was slipping away. We had no idea when or if it would return!

The solution was most unexpected – networking!

Connecting with people on a daily basis to help them helped me more than I can ever say. I set a goal for myself- to meet five new people a day.

I hopped on zoom meetings posting my request "Who would like to book a half-hour zoom meeting, get to know each other, learn how I might help you!" The responses came rolling in!

Those meetings have been my salvation! I have my ability to be of service back! I made amazing connections learning what my others were experiencing. I forgot about the dire predictions on the news, the day's death tolls, and my own problems. I found hope and new perspectives in my new friends' stories.

I was reminded that we have two ears and one mouth for a very good reason! As I listen to their stories, I just intuitively know the questions to ask to learn how I can help. I've found ways to serve others even though we are separated by the miles and the computer screen.

This habit has served me so well. I have moved from feelings of survival to feelings of thriving! The doors will open again. We will go back to face-to-face meetings. I will be taking this new habit into the new post-Covid world!

THE UN-HABIT: HELPING ISN'T KNOWING ALL THE ANSWERS.

Why: It's a common misconception that to help, we have to know all the answers. I spent years believing that I could be of no use if I couldn't tell you the solutions and fear that if I didn't know everything about a given subject, I had no place in the discussion.

This limited my interactions severely because I was only comfortable in conversations with those speaking about something that I believed I knew all about. Eagerly I would listen to the beginning to share their story. Listen, I would say not being the real world as each sentence would trigger a barrage of thoughts. "Oh, I can tell them this. Oh, if only they knew that. When will they stop talking so I can share the solution? Don't they know I already have the answer for them, I would think as I impatiently waited for them to stop talking so I could impart my wisdom.

The know-it-all has many faces: Never letting others say a word. They give advice on everything even before they are asked for it. They are arguing with everybody else's ideas and bossing everybody in the group around. They may be seen to be impulsive, breaking into the conversation before the speaker is done. We question their listening skills due to the fact that they are consumed with what they are going to say in response to what the speaker is saying. They are judged as having an inability to read social cues making the conversation all about them.

The price to all of these annoying behaviors: Missed lessons we could have learned had we only taken the time to listen more. Relationships that never developed because people quickly learned to head the other way when we entered the room.

The façade of know-it-all is worn to cover up feelings of insecurity. Their low self-esteem and fear that their lack of knowledge will be revealed. The mask of the imposter heavy on their head. It's a lonely and isolating life. Knowing all the answers means you can never allow yourself to ask for help or appear vulnerable. The know-it-all feels an ego induced need to be the authority on everything. Seeking to be the center of attention but finding themselves shunned at get-togethers, the last one to be invited to the party. Theirs is the last advice that others seek.

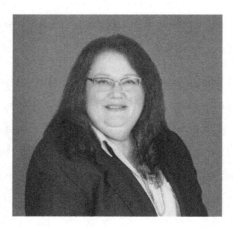

About Brenda: Helps you build stronger relationships, both personal and in your business, by teaching you the arts of listening and questioning. Learn to use your ears twice as much as you use your mouth. Become the person people seek out to discuss ideas and problem solve. Release yourself from the stress, anxiety, fear, and the need to have all the answers. Learn to offer help and receive help with grace and confidence.

24

BE THE CHANGE YOU WANT
CAMI BAKER

Why: When you "Be" the change, you will "Do" the new thing and "Have" the results. One thing is for certain in a post covid world.... nothing is certain. For some, that is a scary place to be, yet there has never been a more exciting time to be alive for others!

Think of the one thing that you feel completely PASSIONATE about that you would like to see change in the world?

The PC (Pre Covid) ways of educating, worshipping, working, parenting, exercising, socializing, farming, networking, and even fundraising are being rethought, reworked, reconsidered, and reborn! Post-covid is the PERFECT time to Be, Do and Have the change you want to see. There is no normal or standard to go by anymore. Once you have thought of a system, strategy, or way of doing things that you'd like to see change, Be that Change!

Do you think children should be taught through life experiences and family togetherness instead of classrooms? Be the example of it and travel with your family in an RV!

Would you like to lead the single mothers' movement of running successful companies from a collective, collaborative center? Be the one who initiates the movement and acquires the center!

Does creating a community where families live together, grow their own food, and become sustainable as a group turn you on? Guess what..... you are not alone. Post covid, these societies will spring up, and it can be you, that is being the change.

Have you thought of a new way to get nonprofits funded by the billions in this post covid world of social distancing and less cash for donating? Oh yeah! That would be me! Our movement of "REAL Agents of Change" have created the system. The best way to implement this change is for us to Be the Change we want in the world by showing others it is possible in our actions.

Now is the time to Be the change. Who can you Be being in this new beginning?

THE UN-HABIT: WORRYING WHAT OTHERS THINK ABOUT YOU

Why: What others think about you is none of your business and will keep you broke and unhappy. Now that the world has been turned upside down, and nothing is normal, what a great time to be "Abbey Normal."

What a great time in history to truly let your "freak flag fly" and just be yourself. Now, obviously, we always want to be respectful of others and never do anything that would be offensive deliberately. However, when we are in constant fear of what others think or being judged by our actions, we simply do not move forward or live life to the fullest.

In a post covid world, we can try new things and new ways of being. We need not be apologetic for how we look, how we feel, or for having an opinion. Does that little voice in your head say things like .... what if I'm not good enough.... what if I'm not smart enough.... what if I'm not dressed right, driving the right car, making the right dance moves or..... or.... what if they don't like me!!??

First of all, others are not thinking about you nearly as much as you might think. You know why? Because THEY are worried about what you and everyone else think about THEM! Secondly, every time you start worrying about what others think, you usually stop yourself from living full out!

I am so grateful that I let go of worrying about what others thought of me a long time ago. I can tell you from personal experience, as someone who taught myself how to hula hoop at 52 and brought people along with me on the journey on Facebook live. Life is a lot more fun when you just show up..... and frankly, people are way more accepting of a few extra pounds or no make-up and of laughing at yourself now in the post-covid days!

So DREAM....... Take chances ..... Make that call..... Post that post ...... Record that video ..... Give that hug ...... Sneak that kiss ..... Ask for that promotion..... Start that business ...... Apply for that loan ...... Dye that hair ...... Wear those bellbottom jeans and stop worrying about what others think about you because you deserve to be happy, do what makes you feel good, and live your best life!

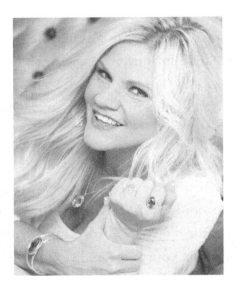

About Cami: Doubling Profitability for real estate professionals when making money and making a difference are equally important. THAT is what the REAL Agents of Change is about. My name is Cami Baker, I am the Charitable Real Estate Strategist who is certifying 1% of Realtors in the Secret Real Estate Niche that is Funding nonprofits by the billions.

25

BE AWARE OF YOUR BODY FUNCTIONS
OLGA BROOKS

Why: During this Covid period, I had hosted my second summit interviewing speakers from all over the world on the topic of "Rediscovering your feminine wisdom and healing powers within. Becoming whole, happy and free". I always get such valuable information for myself even before I interview my speakers. The information I got from Suzen Chang, who wrote a book on healing Lyme disease, had me change my morning coffee habit. Why? Because I love to drink my coffee on an empty stomach for as long as I can without breakfast. Coffee itself is very acidic. I would think it helps people with acid reflux by lowering the production of the acid naturally. But in my case, I know it's not that healthy. It is so essential for our bodies to have a balanced pH. I went on to my own research about it, and this is what I found out.

Our bodies are wonderful, made to create a balance of acidity and alkalinity. Our lungs, kidneys, and brain are playing a key role in balancing pH in our blood. And the brain knows it all. Now, if you don't have problems with your lungs and your kidneys, you are ok. If you have respiratory problems, you get problems with your pH. If you have problems with your kidneys, there is an imbalance with your pH. You are then creating other problems in the body.

Here is a simple explanation. Healthy pH helps us stay healthy. When I learned this, I started putting just a little pinch of baking soda into my first cup of coffee for pH balance and a bit of turmeric to keep my body from any inflammation.

Drink warm water with lemon in it first thing in the morning as it has many benefits. It will create an alkaline environment, plus warm water balances your feminine and masculine energies. Hydrating first thing in the morning and makes your kidneys flush out toxins and function well.

Through our breathing and particularly exhaling, lungs help to free us of excessive acid. What will you do with knowing this information?

THE UN-HABIT: UNHEALTHY ROUTINES

Why: There is one thing that everyone one of us is responsible for; our health. If you have children, they are your responsibility as well.

You can see how important it is to have a strong immune system. Young people don't get sick with Covid or have such mild reactions to it that they barely notice it, or it lasts only a few days.

During this year, I had lost my health insurance suddenly, and that was a bit scary. I stopped working with the elderly because I was concerned about my own health and the people I worked with.

I started by looking into my daily habits. I wasn't consistent with taking my vitamins daily; I changed that. Now I consistently take them, boosting my body's immune system. I've not contracted it even though I traveled to the UK for a book launch back in March 2020 for a book I co-wrote.

It is so important to look into your habits of food intake. Do you read the label when you are buying new and exciting foods? Or are you aware of the ingredients in the boxes you are so used to buying and eating? How about drinks? Are you concerned about what's in the water you consume on a daily basis? How does it compound in your kidneys and liver, and how it affects your other organs and the whole body? I am awake and aware, serving only healthy, wholesome foods to my family and friends.

My journey to awareness of our physical bodies started with the damage to my brain. I am a stroke survivor at the age of 27—the side effect of birth control. I learned the anatomy and functions of the organs of my own body on a deeper level. I had to learn how to walk again. I understand what an impact of even a spec in our brain can do to our abilities to walk, see, find our way home that we take for granted.

Our bodies are our homes. And we need to know that home very well. We need to take care of it better than we take care of the homes (houses) we live in because those homes will outlive us if we don't care for our bodies.

I urge you to look into your Habits and choices of the foods and liquids you consume in your life. Help yourself and your family to make changes by choosing NOT to eat unhealthy foods. Stop consuming what is harming you. And then I am absolutely positive you will make amazing healthy choices that are available and delicious. This will change the course of your life and those around you.

It will protect you from viruses. And will extend your lifespan.

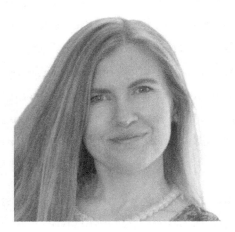

About Olga: My name is Olga Brooks, and I am a Quantum Energy Healer. I create instant release and changes in people's lives by removing all negative energetic influences from their energy field through the Sound Reiki Healing. I teach you how to stay sovereign and protected from future negative interactions and stay free in your high energy state.

Imagine a life where things just flow for you in your business, relationships, and health.

We have been taught many things at home and at school. But not how to recognize negative energetic interferences in our lives. We live for years with the aftereffects of it getting stuck in business, attracting wrong relationships, repeating the cycles where we have been before, blaming ourselves for doing it over and over again. I help you to reconnect with your soul child healing from the effects of childhood traumatic events

26

READ A MINIMUM OF 20 MINUTES A DAY
ALYSSA JERGER MERRITT

Why: Do you have a library at home? Are you like I used to be, buying recommended books but never finding the time to read them? Harry S. Truman said, "Readers are Leaders." We are taught to read in childhood. It is a part of how we learn, expand our vocabulary, skills, input, comprehension, and mostly how to use the words we were learning. If this is how we start out learning, why would we ever stop learning? Today, there are problems with the education system, trying to figure out how to teach all the children and their different learning styles. Some children are lost with the new style of learning. It's most important that part of your child's routine is reading. Now that children are learning online, their comprehension skills are more important. Reading is a cure.

Are you having trouble trying to figure out what to do with yourself now that you are working at home? Is there more time in the evenings? Mornings? At Lunch? Turn off the TV and especially the news. Listen to the news once a day, and do not absorb yourself with the things of the world. Read a book that changes your focus from negative to positive.

Reading is a thing of the present and future. Reading is known to decrease stress, blood pressure, and heart rate. As we find ourselves living in the post-pandemic world, we can find ourselves in a different life. Each day is a new day to begin again. As we grow accustomed to the new world, we need to keep up with our skills. Create a new habit of reading 20 mins a day and see how your mindset changes.

There are so many good books to choose from, starting with the Bible. The Bible is Basic Instructions Before Leaving Earth. Everything comes with instructions in life, and the Bible is ours. Choose books that relate to the season of life you find yourself in. Be intentional with who and what you are reading. This book is perfect for replacing bad habits with good.

Change your input, you change your heart, you change your mind, and you change your life.

During the last year, I picked up reading again. It has helped me change my life and change my business. The average CEO reads 52 books a year. Reading is an exercise for the brain. Mental, Physical, and Spiritual are all of equal importance. Don't stop moving because your life is changing. Embrace the differences.

HAB1T™

THE UN-HABIT: STOP THE NEGATIVE TALK AND DOUBT

WHY: In today's world where mental health concerns have increased to such a capacity that it is mentioned in the World News, negative self-talk and doubt are key factors. Many people today are functioning hurt people who may or may not hurt others along the way. As we have seen with the pandemic, nothing is promised, and nothing is forever, except Faith, Hope, and Love.

Negative self-talk and doubt usually stem from what others have said to us, about us, or how they made us feel during certain seasons of our life. This adds up over time and creates low self-esteem and value, which leads to depression, anxiety, and sometimes self-harm. The increase has occurred because people are living in fear of the pandemic and not faith. It is a matter of your input and focus. Focus on the blessings even during difficult times. Mastering life means you can find the blessing in every situation, even death.

Stop allowing others to hurt you with their words and actions. Zig Ziglar once said, "Don't get distracted by criticism. Remember, the only taste of success some people get is to take a bite out of you."

Get an accountability partner, a coach, a friend, and change your input. Change your focus on the positive and know your best qualities. Do not let the past define you. Change your words, change your actions, and "PPW, prove people wrong," as my friend Israel would say. Get fighting words in your head and when the spirit of wrong thoughts come to the surface, say, "you are a lie, and I choose not to believe you anymore." You are here and have survived the pandemic. Take note and start creating new habits that enhance your life to help others. Before the pandemic, many people struggled and are now dealing with fear, which increases "stinkin-thinkin." Don't let the changes in the world stop you from living in the world with a kind and loving heart toward others. Build each other up.

Be intentional with your words, so you do not cause the same damage to others. "Love thy neighbor" is the most important rule in life. Don't let what is happening in the world rule your life.

Life is what we make it. We are not born with a good or bad life; we create it. Keep in mind everyone is dealing with life changes. Don't let poor mental health be a thing of the future. Have faith and know God is good in all things. Before us, generations have encountered similar downfalls, and those who kept their focus on the right things succeeded and persevered. This is you!

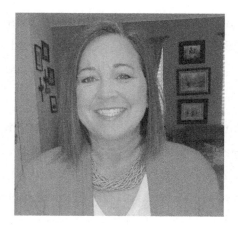

About Alyssa: My name is Alyssa (A LISA) Ann Merritt, and I am here to give you a new lease on life starting with your foundation. Changing your mind and your spirit will give you a different outlook on life. You will get through discomfort while you create new habits. This will make a difference in yourself and many others who will cross your path. You always want to be the blessing, not the lesson. You can find me on Facebook/alyssajerger and Merritt Coaching Group. My husband and I keep the motivation and inspiration flowing throughout the day with faith, hope, and love. "Build the Tribe" is a network of like-minded women who are looking to create change in the world and get us back to the Basics of life by resetting the core values on all levels and every income.

27

FOCUS ON YOU

VERONICA SIMON

Why: You only have one life to live, and wisdom would be to live YOUR life to the fullest without the regret of running out of time. Focus on your priority, of you, instead of other things and people.

As a little girl, I was always encouraged to dream big and not be afraid to pursue my dreams, yet I was taught to count the cost of those dreams and plan accordingly. Though I was supported and never told not to pursue my dreams, I, like many, succumbed to being loyal to others without fully considering being loyal to myself, FIRST. I operated out of the desire to be more of a people pleaser than a pursuant of my dreams.

In my attempt to put myself first, I became an overachiever and trendsetter to outdo and to unfortunately and fortunately drive myself into a private hospital room of solitude. I was too far out of focus that I didn't recognize the error in my thinking. I had overworked myself to prove a point to others about something that I honestly didn't even desire for myself.

The hospital's solitude was where I got to be the focus, just me. There were no other distractions, and I had plenty of time with myself while truly experiencing out-of-body experiences. This is where 'MY' truth became very clear. I was living a life where I wasn't the focus. I was living life while focusing on everyone else but me, which proved to be unhealthy. I had great intentions and aspired to do great things without taking the time to assess ME and 'MY' Why!

While in the hospital and with every attempt of the doctor trying to determine why I was blacking out, why my body wasn't allowing any food intake and not expelling any waste as I was swelling up due to toxins that were being released into my bloodstream. The doctor advised me that if their attempts continued to be unsuccessful within the next 48hrs that surgery would be necessary. Surgery wasn't an option in my mind, as I have enough surgical scars to last me a lifetime.

It became clear to me that I was poison to myself. I was so stressed and experienced hallucinations that appeared extremely real. I knew that none of what I was experiencing was REAL simply because the people I saw are no longer on earth; conversations that I was having or thought I was having with my eyes totally wide open were paramount for my surrender to shift and focus on me!

HABIT

The Un-Habit: Stop wasting time

WHY: Life is not something that honestly is predictable to a degree where one can say that they will have time to do this, that, or the other thing. Neither time nor things are guarantees as we pass beyond 2020 with Covid-19 rocking the world almost instantly into SHIFT AND PIVOT!

Now is the time in which you dare yourself to be a doer, an ACTION taker towards the things that you desire to accomplish, and don't wait until everything is perfect. The truth is, nothing will ever be perfect, nor will YOU! Challenge yourself to take action every day toward things that YOU want to experience. Dare to pursue your dream because only you can fulfill the dream that you desire for yourself. You are the author of your story and the runner of your race (life). Rise up and be the YOU that you desire to be while celebrating every milestone you accomplish because they are the stepping stones to you fulfilling your own desires with you being the FOCUS!

Make yourself the focus and release the efforts of wasting time on what others may want for you. Allow yourself to execute the gift of RELEASING things and people that cause you stress. Stress, my friend, is a silent killer to YOU.

I hope that you lovingly accept these words of wisdom from someone who has been in a posturing position, pleading for a chance to reset and refocus. My ultimate desire is to make me the main thing in my life and a living testament that others may see hope and shift as necessary to be the main thing in their own lives.

Everyone else is taken, so make the best investment of your time become self-aware with the ROI (Return of Investment), which is to "BE YOU, BOO!" ™

To further motivate you, my 15-year-old daughter has inspired me as of late by writing the following quote on my office whiteboard on...

November 1st, 2020, "FOCUS On YOU, Until YOU ARE THE FOCUS!"

Loving You to Life and Beyond, #IAmVeronica

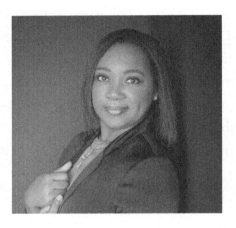

About Veronica: Veronica Simon is the Queen of Corporate Engagement and was the Queen of People Pleasing, who landed in the hospital with serious stress-related health issues, aka CORPORATE & PERSONAL BURNOUT.

I uncovered a better way to live life and wrote my 1st International Best Selling book, "Soul Engagement." Designed to usher you into personal freedom and power, whether in or out of corporate.

What I love most about what I do is giving people hope, especially women. People look at me, my humble beginnings, the child of a teenage mom, and realize that no matter where their starting point is, it can lead them anywhere they desire. Focus on yourself and be INTENTIONAL about living your life. When I am not working or engulfed with my family, you can find me parked at an overlook meditating by the ocean.

28

SCHEDULE THE DAY BEFORE
AARON KONOW

Why: It is great to know what you are doing before you do it. Get in the Habit of planning your tasks the day before. If you want to stay productive with anything, you need to stay focused on the present. If you get distracted by anything, you won't be as productive as you can. When you are doing a task, don't think about the past or the future; think of the present. I have a daily journal that I use for everyday tasks, goals, and quotes. I use a calendar on my phone for everything I do that day, whether it's for my job, time with family, or time with myself. I work with a schedule to stay focused. However, I am open to speaking with anyone during an available time slot on my schedule. I keep at least 1 hour a day for myself. I do something different from most because I check my emails only twice a day instead of whenever I feel my phone vibrate. I also stay focused on the task at hand. Most people don't realize that they are doing it.

I've seen repetitively at stores, restaurants, and at a friends' house, they are on their phone while eating or talking to others. If you are talking to someone, don't be distracted by other things like TV or cell phone. If you go out to watch a movie, you don't need to go on your phone and tell everyone where you are. Don't look up stuff while eating at a restaurant; enjoy your food and atmosphere instead. When someone makes you mad, get it out of your system once and then go on with life. If you stay focused on what you need to be focused on, you will be so much more productive.

THE UN-HABIT: FOCUS ON THE PRESENT

Why: If you get distracted by other things while getting work done, the result won't be as good as if you stayed focused on the task. Always stay focused on the present, be productive, and don't be distracted by other things.

Schedule your workday to remain focused on specific tasks, and you will find the job is accomplished quickly. If you interrupt your task to do another, you may not get back to the first, you may forget.

When it comes to our thoughts;

40% happened in the past.

40% will never happen in the future.

Therefore 80% of thoughts are things from the past or the future that you can't do anything about. That leaves 20%, and of that 12% are things that may or may not happen to you but won't affect you that much. That leaves 8% to stay focused on the present.

A lot of people don't realize that time is your most valuable asset. You will never get any time back. So if you get more done in a specific time frame, you win by having time for other things. Make more home-runs by focusing on the task at hand.

Master one occupation and then work with a task-oriented team of people; it's much better than working by yourself. Minimize distractions during work and work together focused; more will get done, and everyone will have a great time doing it.

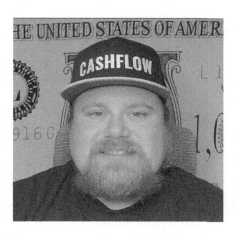

About Aaron: Hi, my name is Aaron, Aaron Konow, the name that nobody can pronounce, Aaron Kon-now. I will teach you the correct way to pronounce my name and grow your Financial Independence.

I'm known as The Wolf of Cash Flow because I help Individuals just like yourself learn to grow their business or start a new business right from home. I help people grow with the money that they make right now and show money management strategies to grow their net worth.

Now I talk to people from their homes on Zoom and mentor them to help grow their financial future. Just so you understand, the two keys to my success is mastering the power of money management and that anyone can do it, even on a small budget.

29

UNPLUG AND UNWIND BEFORE BED

SUSAN LEVIN

W hy: In a world that is shifting, it is important to be able to adapt and pivot with confidence and strength.

What does that mean?

It means that no matter what is going on in the environment around you, taking care of yourself and your health needs to be a top priority.

Unfortunately, we have so many demands and stress during our day—jobs, family, pets, —not to mention finding some time to disconnect, we often sacrifice our sleep. But sleep is imperative for our body to take the time to restore and repair our vital organs. Ideally, a peaceful night of sleep, an average of 8 hours, will allow your immune system, physical health and mental status to function at its optimal level.

Sometimes, it may not be easy to fall asleep or even sleep through the night. Some nights your brain won't shut off because of all your to-do lists, anxiety from the world news or just feeling tense. That is why stretching before bed is one of the best habits to begin!

This ritual allows you time to release tension from the stresses of the day, to lower your blood pressure and to quiet the mind. By creating a nightly habit, your body will begin to prepare for sleep and become tired by the time you get in bed. Just like the way you put children to bed. You create a bedtime routine for their body and mind to signal that it is time for sleep.

Everyone has a different sequence but starting at least 30-60 minutes before the time you want to be asleep is the key. Begin by unplugging all electronic devices. Yes, this means no cell phones or television in bed. Take this time to personally prioritize your self-care by creating this healthy habit.

I personally do 6 key yoga stretches that allow my body and mind to prepare for sleep. This mindful approach relaxes the muscles, unwinds the brain and lets go of all the stresses of the day in order to sleep peacefully. The added benefit of nighttime stretches is when you wake up in the morning, you feel refreshed, less sore and ready for your 5 essential morning stretches that wake up your body naturally and start your day with positive energy.

THE UN-HABIT: Hiding behind the smile

WHY: Have you ever had a smile on your face but all you wanted to do was roll into a ball and cry?

With the many challenges of the covid pandemic, I think we are all suffering with some type of emotional pain and working hard to disguise our true feelings.

To top it off, we are wearing masks that cover all of this up.

However, many of us have been wearing a mask for a long time... before they were the new normal. I understand this concept very well, because I hid behind my smile for years as I went through a horrible divorce. I used my smile as a defense mechanism to protect myself and to ward off basic questions like,"How ARE you?"

It took me 10 years to finally figure out how to stop hiding behind my smile, and accept my life with all its faults. Now, when I smile, it is not a facade anymore but the true meaning from the inside out.

The truth is, I am finally comfortable in my skin and old enough to not care what people are thinking about me.

It took me decades to finally figure this out.

So, I encourage you to stop hiding behind the smile.

Show your true feelings and do not allow the trauma of life to cause you to no longer enjoy the act of smiling.

When you are alone, look in the mirror and smile. Know you are loved, important and matter. Life is a gift to be enjoyed! Smiling brings confidence and allows you to face obstacles.

Tips for an authentic smile:

• Acknowledge your feelings and know it is ok.

• Surround yourself with people who do not judge and will encourage you to move forward and conquer your fears.

• Realize you deserve to be happy.

• Allow yourself to pause and reset.

• Visualize a happy place or someone you love that makes you smile.

• When sad, close your eyes, and take 3 deep breaths through your nose (Inhale for 3 counts of positive thoughts and exhale for 3 counts of thoughts that do not serve you).

• And last and most important, do YOGA.

Yoga builds confidence, balance, focus and the strength to face all challenges and obstacles.

It truly saved my life through the difficult times and allowed me to mindfully remove my mask.

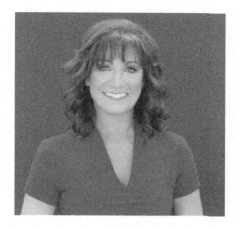

About Susan: #1 Best-selling author, Susan Levin, is the founder of Personal Priorities Yoga and Wellness and has been in the wellness community for over 30 years.

As a Certified Yoga Instructor with a degree in Nutrition, Susan offers a proven online program to help people alleviate pain and strengthen their body through yoga and eating healthy.

Her unique combination of simple strategies only takes 11 minutes a day to give you a lifetime of health.

No outside equipment is needed, just an open mind for the importance of self-care and living your best life with increased mobility, flexibility, strength, and balance.

Susan is known as the Authentic yogi who makes yoga and health fun yet detailed and accessible to everyone.

Learn to adapt to life's challenges with the confidence and benefits of yoga and good nutrition.

30

GRATITUDE FOR CREATIVE EXPRESSION

TESS CACCIATORE

Why: My daily walks, that begins my morning Habit, I look to the skies for the clearing of clouds, I listen for the chirps from the birds, and messages from the crows perched on the phone wires high above my head. I witness the daily messages from nature that give me the inspiration for what I can do to be creatively fulfilled.

Before COVID, I always had my creative juices flowing. However, being held at home, I have had ample time to choose to either wallow in fear, or swallow fear and move into a place of creative expression.

I have found it necessary to do two things: Make a list of weekly projects to stay on track for my overall monthly goals. Then, by surrendering and listening to my creative muses, I let the magic flow. My creative expression fluctuates between writing a story, a song, or a script.

I feel blessed to have many creative outlets. This time of COVID has cemented the process of fully integrating the talents that have been bestowed upon me. Each of us has divine and significant talents that need to be expressed to help us stay focused on the positive; and keep our minds and heart sane in this crazy world.

One of the projects that kept me completely occupied for the past four months was taking our Fifth Annual GWEN Global Luminary Awards to the virtual world. It was important not to let the world's atrocities delay our event, and I needed to heal from the first two months of 2020, where I spent time in Abuja, Nigeria.

I returned home, by the grace of God, just in time for the "lockdown." It took me months to get back on track. When stable again, I achieved something larger than I ever knew was possible, with a three-hour broadcast Concert and Awards Ceremony, bringing artists, humanitarians, celebrities together to celebrate and lay the groundwork for projects in Human Rights and Education.

The satisfaction and pride that I felt when I delivered the project by directing, writing, producing, and editing, I knew that throwing myself into the project would save my sanity and bring me peace to know that there was light at the end of this dark tunnel. The groundwork was laid for the next steps when we can "move about the cabin" and travel again.

Creative expression is in all of us; baking a pie, growing a garden, and laying by the fireplace with a good book inspires us to know that this too shall pass.

The Un-Habit: Overthinking can lead to sinking

Why: Our MIND is a powerful system that can rule our world by displaying positive or negative repercussions to us. There is so much coming at us from all angles in today's world, whether our family and friends or the media, fear-based rhetoric in the masses ready to permeate our minds on a minute-to-minute basis.

So, the habit to break is to not let our minds rule our senses. Instead, we have the chance to follow our hearts.

Our HEART is a powerful system that revolves around intuition, inspiration, and emotional health.

During this time of COVID and beyond, I feel it is important to follow our heart and dive deep into the feelings that take us to the power of love. Love and fear are on the same level, so in every way, we have the choice to react or act with love or fear.

When making a decision or coming out of an overwhelming feeling that can take us to sadness, we need to be cognitive of who we surround ourselves with and what impact we can have on our lives. Whether being alone or with family members, we all have our own sovereign way of being and the power to take our story to a place of positivity.

When our mind chatters away repeating messages of fear and failure, it is important to replace each of these thoughts with the opposite word of being positive.

A good exercise that you can do alone or with a partner is to take a piece of paper and draw a line down the center. On the left column, write down all the negative words and patterns that have been historically trapped in your MIND. On the right column, write down the opposite feeling that shows your HEART's positive side embraces self-love.

Now is the time in our lives to fully embrace self-love and to follow our heart, intuition, inspiration, and let the mind chatter of negativity dissolve like sugar in the rain.

Don't let yourself go to sinking by over-thinking!

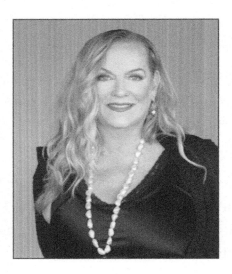

About Tess: Are you ready for a transformation and to fully live your purpose and passion?

Would you rather be stuck in the negative rivers that keep your mind in fear? Or would you rather swim in the oceans of your flowing divine gifts into your creative expression?

Would you rather be trapped in the negative mind-chatter that keeps you in the loop of your past? Or, focus on the heart-centered love that brings all future dreams into the present.

Life is a gift, and we are embarking on a humanity-driven transformation. Now is the time to transform your life into what you are meant to be in the world.

31

DAILY RITUAL WITH YOUR KIDS

JAE MA

Why: Do you schedule out `a dedicated time to nurture your loved ones as you would nurture your work, health, or business? What do you value the most in life? Is it a true connection with loved ones? Is it making an impact? Is it creating wealth? Is it freedom? Take some time to reflect and make a list of these values. What gives you the most joy? If one of the answers to these questions involves connecting with loved ones, then consider creating a daily ritual that is a conscious decision to connect with those you love in your life.

This daily ritual is a token of affection that requires no currency except for the currency of love. It is a simple exchange of energy between two people. Making a conscious effort to connect daily when so many of us are connected to our devices can empower us to recharge our souls. Love is the one thing that keeps many of us going. It is the WHY that can inspire and energize us.

Here is the ritual:

For 7 days, for 21 days, for 45 days, for 90 days, etc. Let us know how this goes for you.

1) Tell each other I love you (verbalize this, write this, communicate this nonverbally, share a token of appreciation). This is also an opportunity to show your appreciation.

2) Give each other a 20 second or longer hug. Connect physically heart-to-heart whenever possible, and stay physically connected for at least 20 seconds. Look at each other in the eye and repeat to them that you love them. If we are doing this over screens, visualize connecting to each other, sending each other love energy through your hands. Send and receive this love you share.

3) Kiss each other on the cheeks. I sometimes kiss my son on his forehead, and I tell him again that I love him.

Once these habits become a ritual, it can become a habit. Enjoy these gifts with all your heart. There will be days when this little extra boost of an exchange of love can transform our day.

THE UN-HABIT: LONG HOURS OF SCREEN TIME

Why: I spent countless hours on screens through Covid as a beginning entrepreneur to empower myself, my family, my friends, and those whom I have been blessed to touch in the world. There were many days where everyone in the household was on screens for most of our waking hours. We developed skills but were disconnected as a family for many hours even though we were under one roof. As the year came to an end, I took the time to reflect. One of the biggest lessons during Covid was learning that we can be knocked down during times of difficulty and obstacles, but we do not have to stay there. It is the lesson of working with whatever we have at this given moment and making it work for our situation and how falling and coming up out of it even stronger. These times of challenges have allowed us time to reflect on our values. At the end of the year, I sat down to reflect after adjusting to being entrenched in these new behaviors of countless hours on screen time. I searched deep within my heart of what my ideal life would look like; it is centered around the people I love and care for in life. This reflection led me to seek answers on how I can get back into the rhythm of balance daily.

Finding time to balance to include those we love in our lives with and without screens can be emotional, psychological, and spiritually crucial in our joy factor. Whatever we focus our energy on expands. Dig deep within your hearts, and the answer will be present itself from within to guide us to the choices we make daily to keep this rhythm of balance. It would be to involve my loved ones more in the activities we do daily.

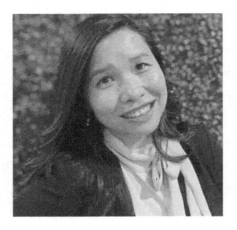

ABOUT JAE: I empower introverts who have felt unseen, alone, or unsupported, knowing they have a voice and message to share to grow and thrive online. Through a simple 5 step system, you will be living a life by design, empowered to empower others online. My mission is to share joy, love, and positivity to leave a legacy in the world. I currently also do this as a coproducer connecting talents and speakers through our Global Talent Show for charity. We recently brought together over 65 talents and speakers for our first 24 hours NYE Show Your Groove Global Talent, collectively sharing positivity and raising funds for two charities given less than 3 weeks to plan this event. I would love and absolutely adore to empower you to grow and co-create with a supportive community online.

32

BE INNOVATIVE AND COLLABORATE
SHEILA FARR

Why: Challenging times provide opportunities for business owners to reinvent themselves and remain relevant and maintain a viable business. It is important to develop a carefully planned and well-executed approach that's innovative. Finding new ways to meet your customers' needs and build your network to share those new strategies can help you become – or remain - a business leader.

We have all been looking for ways to stay connected during the pandemic, and collaborating in business is a great way to do just that. Sharing informative presentations and using diverse panels for interactive discussions can revive stagnant businesses and open the door to new ways to collaborate and broaden one's sphere of influence. It also helps to provide social interaction crucial to long-term job engagement and job satisfaction.

Business growth opportunities often present themselves when you know the right people. One important thing business owners need to be focusing on during challenging times is collaboration. Finding the right person to help share information about your business and products or services can help grow your business by leaps and bounds. This is especially true during a global pandemic when entrepreneurs try to connect and help each other stay afloat. Additionally, with so many people transitioning to remote and on-line working situations, the potential to network across the world has become greater and greater. Collaborating on projects, sharing information and opportunities, and connecting on a global level has become easier than ever.

That's why I recommend focusing on being innovative and networking. Not just by building new, valuable connections, but also by keeping your existing contacts apprised of your goals, progress, and new ways of providing goods or services. Communicating across a strong network of customers and business associates can help you not only survive but thrive in challenging economic times.

THE UN-HABIT: JUST STAY SEATED

Why: For many, life has taught them to play small and "just stay seated" when opportunities come their way. Insecurities, the mindset of lack, and fear of the unknown can cause you to remain chained and paralyzed when it's your turn to stand up and make your move. In life, however, there truly are no magic wands; to be successful, you really must stand up, use your voice, roll up your sleeves, and do the work. Dreaming alone won't make it happen. Wishing won't make it happen. Excuses won't get you any closer to it either. What will make your life amazing is to develop those clear-cut and laser-focused plans to achieve a goal-driven by your passion for it!

You carry within you certain qualities and attributes that contribute to society. You do matter—your life matters. Everything you do has an impact on someone, somewhere, and somehow. When you feel paralyzed by fear and are ready to turn back because the road in front of you feels too unpredictable, take a deep breath, and just begin to move forward one step at a time. I believe we are born with a purpose and a passion for something in life, and that purpose is different for each of us. At the end of the day, who you are, what you do, and how you show up in the world is sacred and unique. Everything you share—whether it's your compassionate heart, your killer smile, your sharp wit, or intellect—has a ripple effect on everyone around you and beyond. You matter in more ways than you might realize. Whoever you are and whatever you do - the world needs you. When you dream big, show up boldly and share your unique essence, you can change lives!

We are equipped with unique gifts and talents that are ours alone, and we are meant to share these with the world. Staying seated and keeping quiet means we aren't living our purpose. For that reason, I say – don't look for the easy way, look out for the opportunities, and when it's your turn – stand up and take it!

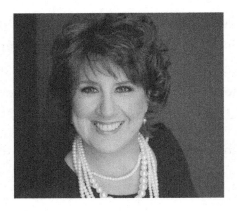

About Sheila: Sheila Farr is an eternal optimist and a passionate business strategist! After 20 years of building and managing million-dollar businesses for others, she stepped out and started her own business in 2017. Now, she's the CEO of Gulf Coast Training & Education Services, LLC, in Biloxi, Mississippi, where she helps struggling entrepreneurs and small businesses overcome obstacles and turn their struggles into success stories. Sheila is a 2-time best-selling author of "Trailblazers Who Lead" and "Courageous Enough to Launch," where she shares strategies and tools to help people propel their careers to a new level.

33

HAPPINESS IS AN INSIDE JOB

DAWNA CAMPBELL

Why: A previous employer asked everyone on a routine basis, "Are you happy?" The question was so frequent when she entered the room; automatically, you started assessing the level of happiness. Many scales for the internal happiness meter were used for measurement when I was approached with this question.

Sometimes I would say "yes," but that brought more questions such as "Are you truly sure?" Other times I said, "Well, I am mostly happy" or "Today I am happy, but yesterday I was not." A favorite response was quantifying happiness, such as, "I am 85% happy," as if happiness could be measured in this way. Avoiding answering this question was not a good choice, either. There wasn't an escape except to deal with my mindset.

Mental notes were taken daily on internal happiness. I quickly realized that the focus was mostly directed at the things that brought unhappiness. Although a natural tendency to focus on what is lacking, subconsciously, I created more unhappiness and unwanted experiences. I was being programmed through life experiences, social conditioning, and the media. My destiny seemed to have an unhappy outcome.

Successful people living an abundant and affluent life have the same questions as everyone "How can I be happy"? They are uncertain how to answer because money was a distraction keeping them in a state of doing rather than being.

One way to discover internal happiness is by keeping a happiness journal. Keep a journal where all the things that brought happiness are recorded. This is a little different than a gratitude journal. Happy moments are recorded rather than thankful moments. This process allows the discovery of the divine essence. Record the happy moments, opportunities of happiness that could be shared. What brings each person happiness is different and a personal journey. This self-discovery process is what allows the divine essence to sing full of joy. When thoughts and feelings are focused on the energy of happiness, you feed yourself happiness. Happiness feeds happiness.

Fill up with happiness, and the outside world will shift and respond to the joy, bringing more.

Wisdom of the Buddha says: "There is no path to happiness; happiness is the path."

HAB1T™

THE UN-HABIT: ANYTHING LESS THAN HAPPINESS IS SELFISH

WHY: Will Smith said: "Her happiness is not my responsibility. She should be happy, and I should be happy individually. Then we come together and share our happiness. Giving someone a responsibility to make you happy when you can't do it for yourself is selfish" in speaking about his wife, Jada Pinkett.

When we allow outside people and circumstances to control how we feel on the inside, we give up our internal power, which is the vice of blame.

Blaming is the allowing of another person, event, or situation to have power over us. Everyone makes decisions and choices in their day-to-day life, and blaming others gives that decision-making to someone else. When blaming happens, it says, "here, take my power, I don't need it."

An example of this is when a parent says to a child, "you make me so ("angry"). In this scenario, the child was given the responsibility for how the parent chose to feel. The child received the blame, and this lowers their sense of worth at the moment.

Blame is not always rational. When an individual choice is made and doesn't work out to the expectation, they tend to blame. Blame is finding fault with someone else or a situation allowing it to steal your natural happiness. Casting blame is a way to self-sabotage and rob yourself of your divine right to experience profound happiness and joy.

Taking the responsibility internally for how you truly feel sets you free. This enables your ability to respond and gives you the true empowerment needed to move you forward to creating.

Everyone is responsible for their own happiness, --- not another person, situation, circumstance, product, service; the environment can do that for you. The expectation and attachment that others are responsible for your choices is pure selfishness when you have the power all along.

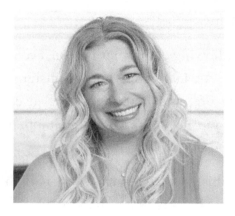

About Dawna: Your thoughts and emotions impact everything that you do in your life. Over 90% of the time, we are completely unaware of these thoughts; and the emotions we have behind the thoughts. How you think changes every day, producing different feelings throughout your body. Sometimes, we find ourselves in a dark space, and we don't always know why.

Dawna Campbell is the author of the book and program, Financially Fit, helping you expose, release, and transform the hidden "why" to empower you to achieve success in happiness, prosperity, and love in all areas of your life. With over 25 years of professional experience, Dawna is a though form leader, a motivational speaker, and maintains an international private practice. Her personal Heart Centered Healing philosophy is to create a world that is a better place for all to live.

34

LET GO AND LET GOD

RONI FRASER

Why: Anybody who knows me personally reading this would scoff: "Let go, let God? Bit rich coming from Roni Fraser; he's spent most of his life arguing against people who believed in God. So, hear me out is what I would say back at them. For most of my adult life, I was an addict. That means that I was the champion of bad Habits. My bad Habits nearly killed me. Literally, I thought I was invincible. I thought I could party like there was no tomorrow without paying the consequences. I was wrong. One day I realized that my parents were going to outlive their only son, my wife was going to become a widow, and my daughter was going to become an orphan. I had to do something. So, I joined a 12 Steps program. The first assignment from my sponsor was to identify a Higher Power. I had to give up control of my own life because that was evidently not working. And I had to surrender my life to this Higher Power completely. I didn't have to turn religious.

I came to realize that we all secretly believe we are God. We think we know best. We think unless we control everything around us, we can never be okay. Paradoxically, the more we strive to control the world, the more we lose touch with it. That truth becomes dramatically obvious to an addict on the brink of death, but it is hard to accept for any 'normal' person out there. Even devout religious people can miss that concept altogether.

You see, faith is powerful. We have faith that no solar flare will zap the Earth into darkness tomorrow. We have faith that the T.V. set won't explode overnight. We have faith that the driver in front of us isn't going to swerve abruptly and cause a collision. Any of these things could happen, yet we get out of the house each morning because we learn to accept that things will turn out okay. And they do!

Then, why not make a habit of practicing your own kind of faith? We trust to accept life as it is. We stop trying to worry, and we learn to live in harmony with the randomness of the Universe. We let go of control and resistance. We have faith in the Universe. We let go, and we let God, confident that things will be okay. And if they're not, that's okay, too. Because it's not up to us, so why worry about it?

HAB1T

THE UN-HABIT: STOP BEING SELFISH

WHY: I know, it seems so obvious, why even mention it? But that is actually the point. We are taught as kids that it is wrong to be selfish. We are shamed and guilt-tripped into being less selfish. The problem is, we aren't taught how to be less selfish or why it is important. It seems obvious, but it is one of the hardest things anyone can do.

Think about it. The truth is that our ego is a very powerful force. We need our ego to survive. Without our ego, we would soon be dead. Quite literally. The ego is indeed powerful. But it isn't the only force governing our thoughts and our actions. We also have a heart. Our heart is programmed to desire a deeper connection with others and share our burdens with them. This creates a conflict between the heart and the mind. There is no need for this conflict. It isn't helpful. Sure, we need to preserve ourselves, but just as important for our sanity, we need to bond with others.

If you have been accused of being selfish more often than you can handle, maybe it means that you are slightly out of balance. The treatment for selfishness is altruism. I'm not saying you should be Mother Theresa overnight. All you need to do is to practice this simple hack:

1. Help others.

2. Commit to help someone else.

3. Listen to their problem.

4. Focus on their need and offer help.

5. Just get out of your head for a moment.

Such a small gesture can deflate your ego over time. The catch is that it has to be sincere. Just do your best to make a meaningful connection. It might feel phony at first, but the payoff is incredible. You will realize that what makes you so discontent, tired, and weary is that we are invested in our own self-obsession too much of the time. It's exhausting. We are so high maintenance! And our ego is such a burden, weighing on us like a ton of bricks.

Just let go of yourself. Focus on someone else. You will be surprised what a liberating experience this can be. You will soon realize that it is in your best interest to stop worrying about your interests once in a while. Win-win!

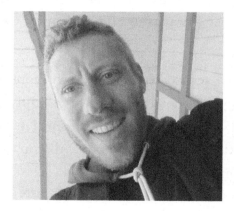

About Roni: Did you know we create our own suffering? Not on purpose, but we do. Crazy, right? We are all a little 'crazy'.

Did you know about the link between physical fitness, mental wellbeing, and spiritual growth? Are you ready to stop suffering and find 'true' happiness?

Read Roni Fraser's free book, Awaken! Surrender, Get Better, Unleash your Power. Learn the ultimate mind hacks for finding 'true' happiness. The author once suffered severe psychiatric disorders and found peace using these techniques. Try them for yourself. This is the product of around 50,000 hours of agonizing research. Roni Fraser did it the hard way, so you don't have to.

Surrender, get better, unleash your power. Awaken from your nightmare, and live.

35

WRITE YOUR GRATITUDES DAILY

TESSA GREENSPAN

Why: When you do this, you get on a track of abundant gratitude, and you begin to flood your mind and heart. As you do this daily, you both exude and invite blessings over again and again. That which you do, you have become one with.

It is so important to be consistent with this activity because it sets the tone for everything -- how you open and close a day. The more you practice this, it will be so ingrained in your brain and heart that you will think about what gratitude means, but you will feel and then emote gratitude.

Brain research has shown how the brain quite literally lights up when we engage in gratitude; there is something magical and specifically healthy that happens. Especially during Covid-19 and how it has captured our attention, health has become more sacred. Isolation has created a unique yearning for the company of others – the physical touch, hugs, feeling the tangible warmth of someone near to us, the eye-to-eye exchange that is so natural, and seeing a smile up close and personal. There is also the absolute pleasure of just simply being in the presence of our family and friends. Sacred.

No doubt that each of us is eager to show our appreciation, gratitude, and thankfulness for our survival. Engaging in this Habit is life-changing because it is mind-shifting and heart awakening.

The beauty of having survived something that we had been so uncertain about is that we become ambitious to move into a more accelerated pace and aim for thriving, which is an ever more substantial and exciting way to experience living. The gift of the virus is that, if we allow it, we have taken this time of isolation from others to recognize how genuinely valuable and fragile life truly is.

At its core of meaning, gratitude is about an all-encompassing connection to that which is sacred, meaningful, precious, and irreplaceable for us. Living in this state of mind and heart is joy-filled, simply marvelous, and that is a beautiful way to do the day, I guarantee it.

THE UN-HABIT: STOP COMPLAINING RIGHT NOW

Why: Once you begin complaining, it is like falling down a long dark hole, a well that you tripped into, and suddenly you are drowning in the cold, dark, dirty water, and there seems to be no way out. You are trapped. There is no visible ladder; the light from up top is almost dim. It is so far removed from where you were just a brief time ago. As you sit there, the water is rising, and your body is frozen in fear, you wonder if these are your final moments, if indeed you are going to drown.

Thoughts are powerful, and they interact with your feelings so intensely that it is hard to separate which are coming from your mind and which are coming from your heart. You are sinking into the mud, and you then begin wondering if you are sinking into worms. Your heart begins to race, and your feelings ask you if you are sliding to the center of the earth, never to return to the planet's surface. Your mind races faster, and you think perhaps you have died, and you are on your way into hell – or maybe you have arrived.

The Habit of complaining takes you on this trip and an expensive journey into darkness. It robs you of your peace of mind and your ordinarily calm rhythmic heart. You are feeling sad, weepy, depressed, and sullen, with no smile available to you. You feel your brow wrinkling and your gut tightening. Your arms and legs begin to ache with tension.

Imagine, if only you had allowed yourself to take the shortcut across the green grass, appreciating every blade of soft green and feeling the warmth of the sun upon your body as your eyes gaze up to the sky and you see the clouds of heaven. You know you are alive. You are breathing. If only you had not needed to complain about – what was it that you felt the need to openly lament over? You cannot even recall it.

The Habit of complaining is just that – it is a Habit, and you have a choice. Your mind and your heart are in your control, not the control of anyone else. Others may have influence, but only you control you. Choose your habits wisely and avoid falling into the well. You can always decide that gratitude is your choice; it is your option.

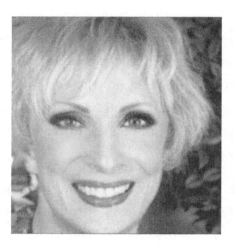

About Tessa: Wake up daily and put that big smile on; it's your best outfit!

36

ASK FOR HELP
BRIAN VANDER MEULEN

Why: During the COVID pandemic, we've had to make more adjustments to our lives than ever before. One of the biggest adjustments was that we have become isolated. One area where this has been prevalent is my willingness to receive when I have been used to giving.

I know this so well because, in the last 90 days of 2020, I've lost my daughter, my dog, and my business partner. As you can imagine, this rocked my world really hard. I have been so used to being in control and steering myself where I needed to go that when these things happened, I was at a loss.

During these difficult times, I have discovered how generous and helpful people in my life have been. I have been repeatedly asked what help I need, and I have learned to graciously accept that help. I have usually been the one to offer help, so this has been an adjustment.

Often, we have no idea what we need until we need it.

It has become more apparent now than ever before that the habit of "Asking for Help" is crucial to forward motion and the foundation for success. Working with people who have strengths where you have weaknesses creates a stronger link in success for all involved.

Even though we aren't physically gathering like before, help is still available, whether it's through a phone call, social media, email, or even a Zoom call. There are some things that even a pandemic can't change, and it's the human spirit of helpfulness. When we feel alone, asking for help is the best thing we can do. Doing this can propel us forward quickly because we get to experience the strengths that others can supply us when we need them the most. Utilizing this habit will only serve us even more as we move through the post-pandemic journey ahead of us.

THE UN-HABIT: DON'T GO IT ALONE

Why: Breaking the habit of NOT asking for help is critical to success in all areas of life.

It is the difference between having the van you need for your special needs daughter and floundering financially to try and figure out how to get her to her needed appointments, not to mention regular travel time with the family.

Not asking for help is the difference between feeling bad or embarrassed for "having to ask," and the power of acknowledging where you are weak and others are strong.

A Chinese proverb reads, "He who asks a question remains a fool for five minutes. He who does NOT ask a question remains a fool FOREVER".

We are so fortunate to live in a time where "HELP" is just around the corner, across a bandwidth highway of light, sound, and wisdom. Help can be sent in the form of a phone call, text message, email, or on a myriad of social media platforms. As I mentioned before, those may be the only options that a lot of us have in the COVID era.

Don Green of the Napoleon Hill Foundation has said this thousands of times, "There are only two ways to get smart; books or to surround yourself with people who are smarter than you."

If you don't know what to do, someone else does. Break the habit of not asking for help and embrace the notion that we are all in this together. There is help on every continent, around every corner, and in the hearts of many.

Break this habit. As Ric Ocasek eloquently said, "Refusing to ask for help when you need it is refusing someone the chance to be helpful." Be the BEST at what you do and help someone else be the best at what THEY do. Swallow your pride if you need to, stand up, sit up, pick up the phone, open the computer app, email or text message, and ASK.

Your life will thank you for it.

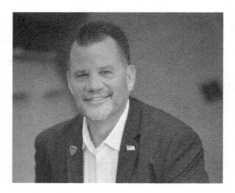

About Brian: As a successful real estate investor/agent, Brian knows the real estate investing in's & out's, both personally and as a coach and mentor. Brian specializes in creative commercial transactions, speaking, and training, where he helps counsel his clients and mentees in ways that will minimize the risks and therefore maximize their returns. Brian's experience in life and business has taught him the importance of teamwork, the power that comes from pushing through life's many struggles, learning to ask for help, and finally having faith and knowing that God is good and always provides.

37

THINK LIFE HAPPENS FOR ME, NOT TO ME

DR. ALEXANDER MANKOWSKI

Why: When something as challenging as Covid happens, it is natural to experience thoughts like, "Why is this happening to me? Nothing good can come of it!" Such thoughts are normal; however, if we dwell on them, they will affect our actions, behaviors, and ultimately our entire life.

When a tornado of life occurs, it may produce enormous upheaval. You may lose a job or a relationship, or when a loved one gets sick, it's hard to see how this can be happening for you. When you are focused on the short-term, what is happening may appear like a loss. But if you take a longer view, what is happening may be EXACTLY what is needed to shake your foundation and bring the hard changes required to get you where you need to be. It all depends on how you frame the situation. Are you going to be defined by the losses you experienced during Covid (what happened to you)? Or are you going to use the lessons Covid taught you to improve your life (what happened for you)?

Life isn't what happens to you, but rather the meaning you assign to what happens to you. This is a choice, even though it may not feel that way. You must ask yourself if what happened is entirely a negative circumstance, or are you assigning a negative meaning to it? What would happen if you looked at the situation from a different angle, from a positive viewpoint? You may be thinking, "How can you say anything positive can come from Covid?" In talking with many people, the conversations always began with the hardships experienced. However, as we dug deeper, people realized many things. They finally had time to honestly examine if They were happy. Time to make closer connections with family, work on personal development/introspection, and found they were strong enough to withstand challenges. The suffering they experienced made them more compassionate, and they deepened their service to others. Would these realizations have occurred without Covid? Honestly-Probably not. Sometimes it takes an event that truly shakes our foundation to awaken our higher self.

Whatever is happening, as frustrating or dispiriting as it may be, is happening FOR you. When you truly embrace this, your life will change. You don't have to like it; it's just easier if you do. Hold to the idea no matter what is going on in your life, what lies within you is greater than any challenge placed in your path. You just have to know that life happens FOR you, not TO you!

THE UN-HABIT: KEEP YOUR PHONE AND LAPTOP CLOSE

Why: We are currently living in the most distracted era of human history. We have access to information instantly and can communicate with people around the world within seconds. Yet, our attention spans have shrunk, and our concentration has disappeared. We may use Covid information as an excuse to use the Internet, but is it truly serving us? The Internet is neutral- it can be used for good or bad. Unfortunately, most of us don't have the self-discipline to be responsible enough to use the Internet! Don't believe me? Check how much screen time you spend/day. I bet it's more than you think. What initially begins as a quick e-mail or check of social media leads one down a 3-hour rabbit hole of searching for GIFs of cats dancing with a hat on. The body has taken over the mind and sabotaged the sub-conscious to focus on things that have absolutely no benefit to our lives.

Scientific studies have found that the average person spends 5 hours/day browsing the web/using apps and checks their cellphone 85 times/day! Yet people's perception of how much time they spend is less than half of that, and they are unconscious of it. Let's be honest, how much of that time you spend using technology is productive? Suppose you spend several hours unconsciously using technology. How can you be fully available and engaged in your work and relationships? It's not just our productivity that suffers. Some of the effects of an unhealthy amount of screen time include: increased stress, depression, anxiety, and decreased sleep quality, enthusiasm, and emotional wellbeing. Our screens are making us sick!

Like every other area of your life, proper boundaries must be placed on your technology usage if you want to be successful. Technology can be a good tool; however, it is also a stress that must be recovered from. Stop using your technology two hours before you go to bed and the first two hours of your day. Spend that time planning, setting goals, and spending time with loved ones, engaging in a real way. It may be hard at first, but the change in your life will be astonishing. If you truly want great relationships with loved ones and yourself, give the gift of your full, unobstructed attention. It is a rare gift these days. Put down the phone and laptop and live. Your whole life will change!

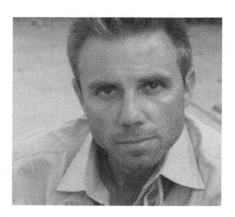

About Alexander: Dr. Alexander Mankowski has been a Chiropractor and Health and Wellness Advocate in Toronto, Canada and Los Angeles, USA. He has mentored professional and Olympic athletes helping them reach peak-performance and success in their chosen sports. He has applied what he learned with elite level athletes and has utilized the same techniques to help others achieve success and prosperity.

He is a motivational speaker and lectures internationally. As a coach, healer, motivational speaker, health and wellness advocate and successful entrepreneur, Dr. Alexander Mankowski has dedicated over 20 years of his life to helping people reach their best version of themselves. His passion is to show people how they can bring their lives back into physical, emotional, and spiritual balance, allowing them to reach their peak potential. He has recently started a production company with several shows in development, specializing in unique content that makes a difference.

38

FLIP THE HUSTLE

DANIELLA PLATT

Why: You Can't Sit On the Sidelines Just Because You're Working From Home.

"Ms. Platt, please pick up your daughter. We are closed until further notice." I zoomed over to her preschool to find a teacher wearing gloves, holding Lysol, with panic in her voice. Next, a text arrived from my husband "effective immediately: NBC employees will be working remotely." When my parents said, you can't visit for Passover; my heart ached: are hugs and kisses canceled too?

It happened in a blink, right? On March 12, 2020, you were hustling, living your normal life. 24 hours later, it all changed? It was very confusing. Weeks later, when broken glass, graffiti, and the national guard filled my beautiful city, I found myself questioning, "am I alive?" How was this happening?

As an action-taker, one who loves warehouses, tradeshows, the fuel of the fast-paced urban jungle, 'going home' was not my game plan. Nor was being with my husband and toddlers in our office, a sanctuary lost to co-working and a playroom.

I share this as each person has a story, a roadmap derailed. What would be the next journey?

What happened next was a miracle, as wonderous as Moses's splitting of the sea! Showing up online were heart-centered entrepreneurs, sailing ships of gratitude, inviting people 'all aboard' to collectively learn to thrive in this new world.

While we wait for science, you must Jump Aboard! It's here where we learned to Flip the Hustle: How do you take different actions to get results?

1. **Practice "Sales Yoga."** Take a deep breath and connect with your community. Keep their mood of mind. Perhaps, they're numb? Or unsure how to plan? Keep it light.

Ask sensitive, simple questions. A favorite question is, "how do you make a PB&J sandwich?" Seemingly silly, you'll be amazed by the reaction. People will relax, giggle, while the answers will be insightful and open the door to opportunities when the time is right. I share more done-for-you scripts in the book *Looking Good.*

2. **Encourage** creators to keep true to their art. When it comes to fashion and lifestyle, your raving fans hunger for your creations. The mentality is "buy now, need now," so adjust.

3. **Gratitude.** Give love. And give more love. Send gift baskets. Create unboxing experiences. Send cards in the mail. Share your roadmaps to success and champion others' success.

4. **Discipline.** When the hustle is your fuel, how can you maintain momentum? To flip, keep to a schedule, and stick to your plan tirelessly.

You are limitless. As you flip, take risks. Stick to your plan. As you shoot for the moon, the worst that will happen is you may land on a star.

The Un-Habit: Stop the blur

Why: When we look back at coronavirus, how will we remember it? Will it be the era of stretch pants? Hoodies? Toilet-paper hoarders? Will you remember Blursday, um, is it Saturday or Tuesday? Or cute family-themed outfits? Beyond the sadness, will you remember days of sunshine? One thing that's certain is you will remember this time as being transformative. And hopefully, you are GETTING DRESSED! Showing up for your day, whether above the keyboard or hitting the streets, it matters!

You see, when you get dressed, you are energized, ready to take on the world, and prepared to make decisions. Clothing is fundamental as to how we are perceived and the energy we exude. Getting dressed affects your mood and sense of self-worth. You light up the zoom house and command attention. You smile at your reflection, and it feels good. Smiling releases endorphins and other brain molecules that fight stress, relieve pain and act as an antidepressant.

You don't sit on the sidelines in your yoga pants! Today, how we work, shop, entertain, and live is through a screen. Now that you are getting dressed, what should you wear?

From Board Room to Living Room: Consider looks that transition nicely from real life to screens. Bold and vivid colors like orange, aqua, and yellow are popular. Remember, your upper body is your on-screen real estate!

Play with Accessories: Have fun with big statement pieces, like chunky necklaces, dangling earrings, or a cool hat. Beading, wooden pieces, and artisanal looks are show-stoppers.

Function & Form: Shop for pieces that are versatile and all-weather to support your year-round needs. During hard times, people crave heritage, cozy pieces, like comfy loafers, clogs, slip-on sneakers, and T-shirts with slogans.

Get Earthy: Boho style, pieces "found in nature" that use natural dyes, have a unique, earthy color or even a 3D texture, or vintage pieces are fun.

Slow It Down: Embrace craftsmanship. Without the fast hustle, shop from designers who share their story and take time to appreciate the little details.

For now, you might still be home. Make sure to have fun. Rock your zoom bod with a nice walk around your neighborhood. Keep a sense of normalcy. The JUNGLE collection of accessories spreads positivity, toting messages of strength and hope. I hope these tips help you get dressed, looking good and help you show up as your best self.

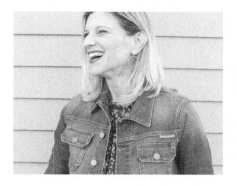

About Daniella: Hi, I'm Daniella Platt. I am known as a vibrant people connector and a Double-A: Apparel and Advertising expert. My mission is to make sure you feel limitless, keep clients loving you for life, and take your message, your art, and your heart to the world.

I work with purpose-driven brands and individuals in three ways: Developing Brand Strategy, Branded and Promotional Apparel, and Sales Coaching.

You can learn to do it yourself: I share how in the #1 best-seller and workshops *Looking Good, Be A Sales Rockstar & Fashion Startup Playbook.* Or let's work together. What I love most about what I do is seeing you flourish.

39

TAKE ACTION NOW

DR. ROBERTA A. PELLANT

Why: There is no time like the present. Turn threats into opportunities. When life hands you lemons, make lemonade. We have heard it all before. But this time, readers, I am urging you to act now. This is the most important habit of success! The international business playing field has been leveled, and we are all are on equal ground. Everyone is basically in the same situation as everyone else due to COVID19 and the effects on thousands of businesses and employees. Some bemoan the fact that business has been awful, so much so that they are out of work. And others who will seize the opportunity to overcome, do, and achieve things beyond their wildest dreams. In 2020, I took the leap of faith to engage in five new business ventures. Three of them paid off, and two did not. The three that paid off contributed greatly to the best year financially in my career, not to mention several accolades and titles that will help with my professional credibility. However, without taking the chance to get out of my comfort zone and pivot headfirst into unchartered territory, I would not have reaped the benefits. For you, it might be as simple as not going back to the corporate world and starting that business you have always dreamed of doing. Time stands still for no one. For some people, all this time might mean going back to school. Obtain a degree that they never had time for before or learning a new language to help increase their professional abilities. Whatever it is, only you can decide to start immediately. Jump right into action now, or at least start taking small incremental steps to help you achieve your goal. Please do not just sit around waiting for a better time than here in this post-COVID world. Time is of the essence, and you will never know what you could have achieved unless you start today.

THE UN-HABIT: PROCRASTINATE AND DO NOTHING.

Why: During COVID19, when most of us 'worked' from home or collected our unemployment checks, many became unmotivated, apathetic even. We found ourselves on social media, in our sweatpants, binge-watching, and streaming the latest shows. And do not get me started on our awful eating habits and lack of exercise and the COVID 19 (pounds) we gained. All these things were newly learned BAD habits causing us to fall out of our so-called normal routines, all because of this virus! We ended up procrastinating and ultimately not doing things that were important to us or stopped doing the things that made us happy or healthy. Our work productivity went down—our motivation to be healthy suffered. We said to ourselves, we will do it tomorrow, and when tomorrow came, we pushed it off until the next day or next week. We must undo this procrastination habit immediately and relearn action steps. We need to institute a new normal on how to get things done and stop the Habits that do nothing for us. I challenge readers to take risks, go outside their comfort zones, push their limits, be creative and dream, and get "DOING." The act of doing is contagious, and it is a habit. Suppose we continue to be indifferent in our day-to-day activities. In that case, we will end up in the same place, the same situation, at this same time next year, or we will find ourselves in an even worse place. The clock is ticking. Break the cycle and do something to change today. All it takes is one step to start or a big move to undo what we have had 10 months to learn. It is time to unlearn what we have learned post-Covid19. What do you have to lose, except maybe a few bad habits!

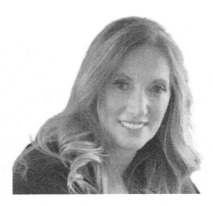

ABOUT BOBBY: Bobby is an MBA Professor of business. She is a co-author of the #1 International best-selling women in business book, Women Who Empower. She is also a co-author in Business Capital 101: realistic expectations for the acquisition of speculative capital, an USGCA publication. Bobby has collaborated on two other 1Habit Books: Thriving Home Office and Writers.

Bobby has started and helped develop two companies: Bum Boosa Bamboo™ a woman ran, certified B-corp bamboo company that was vetted for Shark Tank in 2014 and in 2018 was internationally acquired.

Roberta Pellant Consulting started in 2008 and has worked internationally with both small, high-potential emerging start-ups to Fortune 500 companies. She is passionate about empowering business leaders and their teams to transform their businesses, marketing, and leadership development. She is a certified leadership coach and cultural assessment practitioner by the Barrett Values Centre.

40

GRATITUDE BECOMES A MAGNET

DR. GRACE MANKOWSKI

Why: Gratitude enables individuals to live in the present moment caring for others and themselves and having a positive outlook towards life. During COVID-19, it is easy to get caught up in fear, negativity, and worry for our loved ones and ourselves. The horror of people dying on their own without being able to be with their families was something that extremely upset me. To deal with all these new intense emotions, I started a gratitude journal.

Individuals, who have a gratitude practice, are said to be happier and have a deeper sense of their world. There's a reason gratitude is an integral aspect of countless spiritual traditions and central to many religions, including Christianity, Buddhism, and Hinduism. The benefits of practicing gratitude are nearly endless. People who regularly practice gratitude by taking time to reflect upon the things they are thankful for experience: more positive emotions, sleep better, feel more alive, express more compassion and kindness, have decreased cortisol levels, decreased stress levels, increased serotonin and dopamine in the brain and an increased immune system. Having gratitude for positive events has a twofold effect; it directly increases serotonin and indirectly keeps you from remembering negative events. Scientists found that, like Prozac, gratitude can boost the neurotransmitter serotonin and activate the brain stem to produce dopamine. Feeling grateful increases your brain's production of dopamine, which is the feel-good neurotransmitter. People with low dopamine have impaired thinking, memory loss, slowed reaction time, depression, and lack of motivation. Scientists also found that when we are practicing gratitude, this increases the activity in the hypothalamus. This is important because this part of the brain controls essential bodily functions such as eating, drinking, and sleeping. It has a huge influence on our metabolism and stress levels. Improvements in gratitude can have wide-reaching effects such as improved sleep, decreased depression, and having fewer aches and pains.

Thinking about how you could be grateful sparks your brain activity, critical to sleep, mood regulation, and metabolism. Just the act of searching for gratitude is beneficial. The principle of Hebb's Law states, "neurons that fire together wire together." The more we think about gratitude, the more our brains will wire that way. Thus as our brain becomes more positive, we will attract more positive situations, thoughts, and people towards us like a magnet.

THE UN-HABIT: ASKING PERMISSION TO LIVE YOUR DREAMS.

Why: COVID-19 has resulted in many people having the time to turn inward and assess if they are truly happy and living their best life. Many have concluded that they fell into the "rat race" and are not following their passions. I have a friend who is a highly successful entrepreneur. Throughout his career, he's had hundreds of people ask him if they should go into his industry. He tells every one of them the same thing: that they shouldn't do it and he tries talking most of them out of it. The interesting thing is that in most cases, he succeeds. Watching this surprised me, and I asked him why he does this. His answer was, "Those who are going to succeed will do so regardless of what I say, and if it is their true passion, nothing will stop them."

No one will ever give you permission to live your dreams. If you need permission to do something, you probably shouldn't do it. As children, we had the protection of our parents. That protection meant that we had to ask for permission to do things. Suppose you find that you're always procrastinating, waiting for more information, or waiting for advice. In that case, you need to ask yourself if you are just asking for permission? And if you find that you are, you have to take a step back and realize that you're in charge. Advisors are great, and they can teach you to steer clear of things that you shouldn't be doing. The best advisors don't have a vested interest in your business, and that independence keeps them objective. In the process of building and running your business or following your passions, you're going to have to make a lot of decisions. Getting advice is critical, but you have to make the decisions and take the glory or the blame in the end. Remember, you don't need permission; take advice but act on your own. Follow your passions because life is short. You don't want to reach old age wishing you dared to do what your heart really wanted.

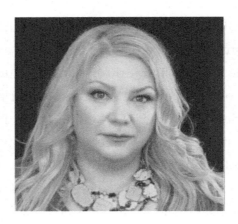

About Grace: In her global humanitarian work, Dr. Grace Mankowski has developed the program Civility Interruption Strategist that helps one uproot destructive patterns in mankind, releasing them to live a free and joyous life. Dr. Grace Mankowski is an International Best Selling Author, International Motivational Speaker, Chemist, and Doctor of Chiropractic. She was a Professor at Seneca and Centennial College, where she taught Business and English for several years. She has worked with Olympians, professional athletes, actors, and CEO's of companies, inspiring them to be the best versions of themselves. Her specialties are designing nutritional, detoxification, and infertility programs. She has helped many abused women and Indigenous people with her

Dr. Grace Mirror Method ™. Her humanitarian initiative has now evolved into a global movement where her work is particularly focused on developing countries and at-risk communities.

41

DO ONE THING DIFFERENTLY DAILY

JEANETTE ERIKSSON

Why: Covid-19 has created an even more unpredictable world than the one we lived in pre-2020, in which we all must continue to live comfortably and ideally thrive in. New ways of living demand new ways of working. New ways of working create new ways of living. Life is a flowing medium, and we need to flow with it. Like a business that becomes stagnant due to inflexible leadership and without innovation, our minds need to change and flow - to create but also to cope. Coping mechanisms derive out of how you look at situations. If you are open and flexible, your solutions will be too.

By staying at home and even professionals secretly wearing PJ's during meetings, we remain comfortable in our concern, safe, and full of 'hygge,' which helps us feel better in our newly created world. This comfort also means we slowly become less flexible and 'change' slowly start to scare us, which is the total opposite of what we need to thrive in a post-Covid world. They say that "you can't teach old dogs new tricks," and what was earlier reserved for the older generation is now starting to affect many of us, of all ages. All society members are at risk of staying in a comfort zone, sticking to small-world routines, which does not create exciting new solutions or make us grow as individuals. My advice is: change it up! Start small by getting into the habit of doing one thing differently each day.

Start with setting small challenges at home by doing a simple daily task differently or trying a new approach to an everyday event. This will kickstart your brain into processing differently, and before you know it, you, as a leader, entrepreneur, partner, will utilize this skill in every bit of your thinking. Outside of the box, forward planning, continuously pondering what you can do (better) with what you already have, but also easily discovering new ways to create from scratch. The Covid world is an unexpected one, where things continuously change. This will set you up to roll with the punches – and being successful whilst doing it.

Trust me, gradually, uncertainty will not be as scary anymore, and instead, you will rise to whatever challenge life throws you in your post-Covid life - with innovative solutions and a stronger mental attitude. And before you know it, you will proudly treasure the sudden ability to conjure up 'dinner' out of mamma's lingonberry jam, leftover lasagna, saffron buns, and a pile of rocks.

HAB1T™

THE UN-HABIT: CONSTANTLY BEING AVAILABLE

WHY: The online meeting platform is loudly pinging from the improvised home office. And pings again. And now it is ringing, which feels like hysterical and frustrating nagging. Isn't it typical? You have diligently sat at the computer all morning in back-to-back meetings and finally managed to go to the kitchen to make a cup of coffee and have a little breather. When you return to your workspace, the screen is full of messages and missed calls. And for every 'chase', your heart sinks a little bit further, and the feeling of 'unavailability-worry' wins over reason, which should simply be the entitlement of taking a screen break or simply a loo break. So, you quickly message back explaining why you were not available, and back in the constantly-available-online hamster wheel you go.

In our now uber-online-developed world, there are many forms of communication where you need to uber-present. Now is the time to streamline your work responsibilities to manage it all and set some online boundaries and build trust to work without being 'seen' by constantly being online. A friend recently described how her 7-year-old accepted an incoming online call 2 hours before work officially started. The result was suddenly being presented to the CEO in inappropriate sleepwear and crazy hair. The point here is not that the child was too computer savvy to create an awkward situation, but that 'online boundaries' had not been set. For many, the workdays do not only start earlier than planned, but the unstated expectation of being available continues into the late evening. Which, in practice, means you end up being constantly 'at work', never feeling like you can fully relax.

So, how do you avoid this stress-inducing downward spiral? It is simple. You make yourself unavailable. I am not advocating disappearing from the work grid and getting into trouble. Instead, I suggest having an open and honest conversation with colleagues and bosses, agreeing on what is expected and acceptable. Encourage discipline with regular breaks and 'time-outs' in your day, as these can be invaluable in helping you pause, re-energize, and refocus with clear start and end times, where you can feel comfortable totally logging off. Make your availability in your working hours clearly set out. A Healthy Habit for everyone to participate in and understand the benefits, and then fully commit when it is 'on'-time and then be your best 'logged-off' self.

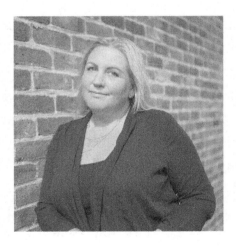

About Jeanette: Jeanette Eriksson created Nordicly (Coaching and Consulting) out of her passion for making people and systems work and feel better. Jeanette's outstanding personal skills, system improvement knowledge, and understanding of the benefits of great coaching derive from 15 years of people and project management experience. Having led large teams at a major London university for many years, whilst gaining national sports success, both as a captain and player, and at management level, Jeanette has learnt all the tricks of the 'personal and business development' trade. So, suppose you want your processes and systems improved. In that case, you need assistance with new and innovative Scandinavian thinking, or you need help to build your people and help them achieve clarity and progress in life and/or perform at a higher level at work, Jeanette is your Nordic(ly) solution.

42

BE GRATEFUL EVERY DAY
MARY ELAINE PETRUCCI

Why: "Cultivate the habit of being grateful for every good thing that comes to you, and to give thanks continuously. And because all things have contributed to your advancement, you should include all things in your gratitude."— Ralph Waldo Emerson.

COVID-19 has turned my world, like yours, upside down. I decided that I would be grateful for the friendships that I cherish, things that I own, and what I want to create in my business. I am using prayer to connect me to God, who knows how to have me live my best life to serve others.

I totally agree with Ralph Waldo Emerson's quote above because I have had many experiences that have been life-changing, and I am now beginning to see how gratitude can influence my life for the better. Gratitude awakens and allows me to be more present in my life so that I can impact others' lives by being more my authentic self.

Scientists believe that gratitude is more than feeling thankful. It's a deeper appreciation for someone or something that produces longer lasting positivity in one's life. I am now intentionally and consciously recognizing the things that other people have done for me. Gratitude provides me the opportunity to connect and establish a closer relationship with God. This shows me the many tangible and intangible ways that He provides me to serve others' needs.

Regardless of outside circumstances, gratitude makes me more resilient while launching my business. It strengthens my personal and work relationships. It allows me to make improvements in my health, reducing stress and worry. Being thankful provides me more determination and energy to complete critical tasks daily to achieve personal and work goals.

Developing an attitude of gratitude allows you to enjoy the small joys that occur each day on your life journey to achieve your greatest accomplishments.

THE UN-HABIT: DON'T BE UNGRATEFUL

Why: "We can only say that we are alive in those moments when our hearts are aware of our treasures." Thornton Wilder

Being ungrateful for the things you have or what others have done for you declares that you are or want to be self-sufficient and deserve something when you didn't earn it. You use others to achieve what you want by constantly requiring others to satisfy your needs and desires without regard to how others served you. You always expect people to do special favors for you with no need to pay back or pay forward.

Because you cannot appreciate life as an amazing gift, you become dissatisfied when people or experiences don't live up to your standards. You have unrealistic expectations and frustration where you are unable to appreciate the positive experience or interactions with others.

You are never satisfied with your accomplishments and are always looking for another goal or position to achieve. You are resentful of what happened to you in the past. You have a sense of entitlement of what is owed you and continually play the victim. You only reach out to others when you need assistance; however, you don't let others ever forget that they didn't help you in a specific situation. You have no genuine concern for others.

Ingratitude eventually impacts your interactions with others, creates physical and mental health issues, and prevents you from seeing/enjoying the beauty and goodness all around you. Your behavior now becomes your prison, and you start to blame others for your isolation. You don't realize that you created your own' prison.' You live on an island of despair, offering you misery because you can't get what you want.

You have a choice to make today. You can be ungrateful and live a miserable life by using others to achieve what you want or be grateful for all the wonderful goodness around you.

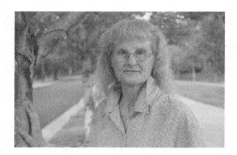

About Mary Elaine: I'm known as the Baby Boomer Healthcare Advocate because I provide access to leading healthcare information from thought leaders in traditional and alternative medicine. I also launched a podcast called Boomers on Fire, where I interview health and wealth experts about concerns that Boomers have about living their legacy.

I am a Speech-Language Pathologist who successfully diagnosed and treated children and adults to give them a 'voice' to communicate their wants and needs. I also met and exceeded sales quotas for neurorehabilitation, home care, and pharmaceutical companies. I am the author of the upcoming book, "Forever Exhausted?" But it wasn't always like this. My family legacy starts with a strike in the coal mining towns in Southern Colorado. My grandparents lost their oldest son because they were refused access to healthcare and their remaining 3 children perished in the Ludlow Massacre. My younger brother was accidentally electrocuted at 15. So now, I have decided to dedicate my life to helping you revitalize your health, wealth, and legacy to lead your optimized life.

43

TAKE THE WALK
MARGRET JONS.

Why: You need to take the walk to go to make your life greater than it has been. Every step of the journey that you take. It will lead you to a different place, not only will it improve your health. It will create a strength in you; it will also give your time to enjoy nature if you're able to go there for a walk.

Sometimes we need to take the first step to be able to go to places that we didn't dream of. It could also be the first step through your own fear.

For nine years, I have been taking a daily walk. On that walk, I have been listening to positive motivational speakers; I've listened to books. I have trained my mind to stay as positive as possible.

I can truly tell you that I have to walk to my health again. I was overweight, with high blood pressure, high blood sugar, and lots of pain. I didn't have any strength in my body because I almost gave up on life. But I decided to take the first step of going outside of my comfort zone and walk towards my health, life, and happiness. If you can't get out of the house, walk around the house listening to your favorite music. Listening to your favorite books. Listen to more motivational speeches. Just move a little bit.

It also might help you just dance a little probably no one is watching anyway.

THE UN-HABIT: THERE IS NO DISCOUNT

Why: Life will never give you a discount. You may ask for it, but there isn't one. If you stop procrastination and you do the little things that you have been planning to do. Then maybe you will half a discount on the guilt that you were otherwise always beating yourself up with.

Guilt and shame, those feelings will give only give you a discount on the quality of your life. Shame is the feeling that will tell you that you're not good enough. Being workable will give you freedom. You might not feel it, that right away, but if you choose to stand tall with a strong back. And a soft front but always keep the fire of life in your heart and be able to embrace the challenge, the difficult, the fights life will throw at you then, my dear friend. You are not taking any discount.

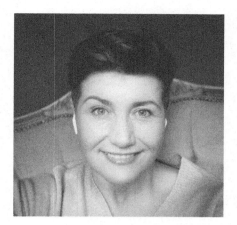

ABOUT MARGARET: My name is Margret Jons, a life coach. I am known as the woman who works in life with joy and motivation because I have walked away from 120 pounds of being overweight and depressed.

Now I help people find their journey and walk their path to success and step into their greatness.

I grew up in Iceland, where the northern lights kiss your cheeks on the long winter nights. My mission is to help people to find the courage and take the walk they have to take. I love seeing people straighten their back and embrace life with no discount.

44

TO SEE THE BLESSON IN EVERYTHING
LAURIE K GRANT

Why: This an essential habit to acquire to live your life in a state of calm or peace. As you progress through life, you will have many experiences. Some you may consider challenging, while others you may consider fruitful and rewarding. However, if you look at life from a spiritual perspective, there is no duality, there is no good or bad, there is just the reality of now.

No experience in life can really be considered as blessed or tragic – it just is. If you refer to the Tao story of the farmer, each time his community tells him an event is blessed or tragic, he responds, maybe. All the events or experiences in your life carry both a blessing and a lesson. Sometimes you will not recognize either one or both of these until much later in your life. The realization may not show up until you change your viewpoint or perspective on how you perceive the experience. You can change those as often as you choose.

Many people believe their thoughts represent their reality and are unique to them. However, we have a conscious flow of universal thought patterns that move from one brain to the next in the energetic state. You are not responsible for each thought flowing through your brain; however, you are responsible for the thoughts you choose to live in your brain. It is these thoughts that bring you your perspectives or viewpoints on what you experience in life.

Living with the mindset of seeing each experience as a "Blesson™" lets you observe the ebb and flow of life instead of having a reactive or proactive approach, which allows you to live your life in a state of calm or peace. This will enable you to be open and curious about what life brings, rather than reactive and resistant, which could mean missing opportunities. When you can live in this non-attached state, you receive and appreciate both the blessing and the lesson in everything you experience or, as I call it, the "Blesson™." You are indeed living in NOW, which is the only moment you truly have to be focused and aware of.

THE UN-HABIT: STOP LIVING IN YOUR PAST OR YOUR FUTURE

Why: "If you are depressed, you are living in the past. If you are anxious, you are living in the future. If you are at peace, you are living in the present."

Lao Tzu

Some people live in the past because they don't or can't cope with their present circumstances. Others do so to avoid the fear of what may come in the future or are stuck on reliving a traumatic event (victim state) repeatedly.

Losing the experience of now is what happens when you live in the past. You are borrowing precious time from yourself and missing out on present opportunities. Yes, you may need to look at the past to understand and process an experience to learn, heal, and grow, but you do not need to live there. Wishing for what might have been or replaying familiar and comfortable memories is taking you away from creating in your present moment.

On the reverse or other side of living in the past is worrying about the future. You are worrying about things that have not happened, and more than likely will never happen. When you worry about the future, visualizing a negative outcome, you're living in illusion as you cannot predict the future. This serves no purpose except when it moves you to develop positive goals and plans.

You cannot control the future; it is governed by unpredictability. It is the nature of life, so it is unrealistic to think you can control your future. By living in a constant state of anxiety about the future imagining worst-case scenarios, you're surrendering your personal power to create for your life.

Your past is gone, you can't change it, it's gone. Your future does not exist, and you can't predict it; it's not here. The only place you can be is present right now in your life with no regrets and no expectations. Living in the here and now will give you improved mental, emotional, and physical health, in other words, peace and calm.

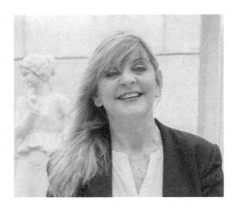

About Laurie: Laurie K. Grant is a digital designer designing since ARPANET birthed the Internet in the early 90's. She is the creative genius behind SHYUI, delivering Effective Messaging for Success! SHYUI provides Digital Transformations that are modern, clean, efficient, and cost-effective. SHYUI uses 3M Web Design - Mobile, Modern, and Minimalist combined with Content Magic to bring your business vision to life, making you stand out from the sea of sameness. In today's fast-moving marketplace, this provides your business a digital advantage while stimulating business growth by increasing awareness of your brand, products, and services.

45

STACKING A NEW HABIT TO A DAILY ROUTINE

MARIA LUCASSEN

Why: In real life, you come across new Habits that you like to implement all the time, but often they do not last very long. You might do them a few days in a row, and maybe even a week. But then life takes over, and you forget about the Habit; this is what often happens. Still, when you intentionally create a new Habit and stack it to something you do already daily, you are triggered to do it when the automatic Habit shows up on your daily schedule.

For example, I used to go to the gym a few times a week, but during the pandemic. I didn't go as I was scared to get the virus. After a while, my body showed signs that I was not taking care of it as I used to. I changed my daily routine to add specific exercise daily.

I didn't have time for 30 minutes, so I divided it into 3 x10 minutes. In the morning, after I finished my meditation, I added a routine of six different short movements to strengthen my core. Stacking here is: when I finish the meditation, I get up and do the exercises. In the evening, I was waiting for the tea water to boil, so I added in to use the spin-gym for 5 minutes. Stacking means: when I put the cup with water in the microwave, I get the spin-gym equipment so I can be ready to start when the tea is brewing. The other 10 minutes are during coffee breaks and lunchtime: when I make a break for the restroom, I will go outside and walk around the building. If I do this five times a day, I add another 10 minutes and many steps. You can also walk the stairs or whatever area inside or in the garage. Just stack it! You probably can find more time slots to add a task, i.e., do the spin-gym exercise while watching the news on TV. Also, certain physical activities, you could add some 'brain' workout. Say, when you are cooking, you could listen to a book on audio if you would like to read more but don't have the time to sit down.

You can reward yourself with small pleasures such as your favorite tea. After a month of doing it consistently, treat yourself to a new workout shirt.

THE UN-HABIT: STOP CHECKING YOUR EMAIL CONSTANTLY

Why: You get more out of your day if you do not get distracted by opening email all the time. You can focus more on the activity that you are doing and complete it in a shorter time frame.

For this to work, I set the timer of my Kitchen alarm when I am at home to give me 30 minutes to do my email when I start the day, again after my lunch break, and before I finish for the day. It works great to focus on more critical projects with my full attention and get these done efficiently and effectively.

When I look at my inbox, I quickly scan the sender's name, looking for my boss or a person who has a high position in the company; those I will answer first. And when I get a message outside the Email reply blocked timeframe, I still look at it to see if it can wait till the next email allotted time.

Working from home where I was watching my business email and my job email on two laptops, I spent too much time on this kind of activity, which interfered with my work and business productivity.

Another way to be more organized in your email response process is to use categories and colors. At a certain time of the month/quarter/year, recurring tasks are creating email messages. Decide on a color code for the different categories, and file them in the correct folder to not crowd your inbox. Once done with the specific task that you received the messages for, remove the category so you can use it again for the new batch to come in.

Lastly, if your email system allows, set up rules for messages that you need to keep but do not have to look at until you do a monthly or quarterly report. The system will immediately file it in the correct folder.

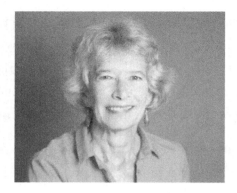

About Maria: Maria Lucassen is a highly experienced corporate career junkie who worked for over 40 years. She has a passion for helping career women shift their perspective on creating and living a blissful retirement after leaving their 9-to-5 job.

She is the CEO of Maria Lucassen Coaching and is seen as the go-to expert for anyone who wants to transition out of corporate employment. She organizes workshops for women who are ready to plan their retirement, helps them individually or in groups to prepare for a happy next phase in life that is fun, purposeful, and affordable; Maria helps them rock retirement and have the lifestyle that they want

Her coaching approach is compassionate, practical, and results driven. She is a resourceful and open-minded problem solver and dynamic supporter for career women who choose to enjoy a new liberated, and meaningful life.

46

ADJUST YOUR FOCUS, EXPAND YOUR HORIZONS
MICHELE MARSHALL

Why: Through mindfulness practices, you can clear the fog caused by feelings of stress, strain, anger, anxiety, sadness, and fear. I encourage you to take on some of these activities to make way for a positive perception of yourself and the world around you.

Adjust Your Focus

What you focus on grows. Choose to focus on what you can control - your attitude and your response. Develop a hopeful attitude and appropriate responses. Shift your perspective to the activities, resources, environment, communities, and people that contribute toward the betterment of yourself and those around you. The ancient text encourages us to focus on the honorable, noble, right, pure, lovely, admirable, and praiseworthy matters or things. Set your thoughts on what serves you and how you can add value to others.

Expand your Horizons

Take an online training course to learn a new skill or build upon a current skillset to advance your career or business. Take on a new hobby such as learning to knit, sketch, play a musical instrument, write poetry, or gardening. Learn how to use graphic design software or video editing. Learn to speak and write in a new language. Expand your horizons and, most importantly, apply what you have learned. While knowledge is power, applied knowledge is freedom.

As an essential worker, my work demands have increased while resources are limited. It became vital for me to make these practices a Habit. For me, this Habit has blossomed into a firm resolve to create a clear perspective built upon hope, instead of panic, while finding a community where I can flourish while adding value.

I encourage you to take on some of these activities for yourself. You will find by incorporating these activities, you have created a serenity for yourself amid a time when others may say the opposite exists.

THE UN-HABIT: SELF-MEDICATING

Why: Let's step in front of the mirror of self-medicating and see if you recognize a bit of yourself in the reflection.

Do you appear strained from information overload on the number of covid cases and untimely deaths? Are there signs of stress from home-schooling or figuring out remote learning for your child? Financial stress for job loss? Are you overwhelmed by job tasks and projects? Has the temperament of others cause you emotional pain?

Feelings of stress, strain, anger, anxiety, sadness, and fear can trigger the need to find a coping mechanism to distract or escape that feeling. This dangerous Habit can cause even more significant problems than the source of those provoking feelings.

If you're an emotional eater, you might self-medicate with food as a way to suppress or soothe negative emotions.

If you want to counter the feelings of sadness or anxiety. You might self-medicate with alcohol, psychostimulants, caffeine, cannabis, opiates or opioids,

Suppose you want a distraction to take your mind away from those provoking feelings. You might self-medicate with financial-based distractions such as online shopping, online gambling, or gaming.

These methods of 'escape' may seem manageable at first. However, as the occurrence of the provoking feelings become more frequent-the use of self-medication also increases. The compounding effect of one or more of these modalities will eventually impact your daily life. Negative repercussions for yourself will include becoming overweight, unhealthy, substance abuse, and addiction.

This damaging pattern can then overflow to negatively affect your relationship with family, friends, and co-workers.

Upon gazing into the "mirror of self-medicating," if you recognize yourself, I encourage you to take the necessary steps to cut back on your frequency (or doses).

For me, it was around Day 30 of lockdown when I noticed I was consuming three glasses of wine daily to calm my nerves. At that point, I recognized I could potentially spiral into a destructive pattern. I've cut back on my consumption. I even saved some money in the process.

Seek the necessary layman or professional guidance toward healthier coping mechanisms.

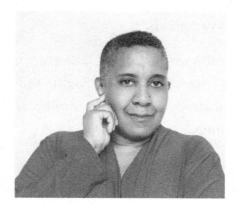

About Michele: As an essential worker, I understand the challenges of our post-covid world. The day-to-day matters to ensure systems and services are functional to allow 200+ administrative staff to work safely from home has sharpened the skills I acquired in my 25 years of experience in the customer service industry. However, the growing work demands made it necessary to maintain personal safety and sanity. Knowing the power of effective Habits, I formed a new Habit that has allowed me to thrive.

47

DRINK A MINIMUM OF 64 OUNCES OF PURE WATER DAILY

DAVID MEDANSKY

Why: Was COVID 19 your wake-up call to improve your health?

One Habit to improve and change post-COVID is to drink more pure water. Drinking more pure water is a Keystone Habit. A Keystone habit is changing one Habit that can change your entire life because it has a ripple effect.

Water is extremely important for maintaining good health. Our bodies are comprised of 60 to 70 percent water. Yet, more than 75 percent of the U.S. population suffers from chronic dehydration. Plus, more than 71 percent of the U.S. adult population is overweight. There is a correlation because much of the time you when you think you're hungry, you are thirsty. This could be one reason most of us overeat. We should be drinking more *pure* water.

This means if you changed one Keystone Habit, such as drinking more pure water and giving up soda or diet soda, you might have more energy, feel better, improve your health, and lose weight.

In my opinion, pure water is distilled water, water processed by reverse osmosis, or spring water. It is not processed flavored waters. There is a debate and dispute about which is better between distilled water, reverse osmosis water, and spring water. You choose which is best for you.

How much water should you drink each day?

That depends on which expert you want to believe. Some health experts recommend you drink a minimum of 64 ounces of pure water each day. Others suggest you drink one-half of your body weight. For example, if you weight 200 pounds, you should drink 100 ounces of water each day. And if you do strenuous physical work or exercise a lot, you need to drink extra water.

COVID caused many people to gain weight. It is referred to as the "Quarantine 15" because many gained between 15 to 30 pounds during the quarantine.

The BIGGEST mistake, however, to lose weight is going on a diet. Some studies show that 95% of people fail diets. That is because diets are designed to fail. They tend to be extreme, temporary, hard to stick with, and potentially harmful.

So, in my opinion, the 1 Habit to pivot your life in a post-COVID world is to get in the Habit of drinking more pure water, preferably at room temperature without ice, because it will help improve your health.

T<small>HE</small> U<small>N</small>-H<small>ABIT</small>: S<small>TOP DRINKING SODA OR DIET SODA</small>

Why: It is important to break the bad Habit of drinking soda and diet soda because they cause weight gain and other harm to your body. Here's why.

Our bodies are comprised of 60 to 70 percent water. Not soda or diet soda. You wouldn't feed your dog or other pets soda or diet soda? Of course not.

The primary reason not to drink diet soda is that it contains Aspartame. What this means for you is that there are 92 documented adverse side effects of Aspartame. One of them is that it causes people to gain weight - *not* lose it. Aspartame affects your metabolism, so you cannot burn calories.

While diet soda may contain zero calories, it will prevent you from reducing weight and cause you to gain weight. It also inhibits or prevents your body from absorbing vitamins, minerals, and other essential nutrients. That is why it's dangerous. You are depleting your body of the proper nutrients, and it goes into starvation mode, which causes weight gain. Further, Aspartame increases your cravings for sweetness. What this means for you is you crave sugar. Just because Aspartame is legal does not mean it's safe.

You should avoid drinking soda because many sodas contain High Fructose Corn Syrup (HFCS). HFCS is a sweetener processed from corn starch. High fructose corn syrup is linked to obesity, diabetes, and even some forms of cancer.

Manufacturers use high fructose corn syrup because it is much cheaper and easier than producing sucrose (ordinary table sugar.) High fructose corn syrup and table sugar both have four calories per gram.

High-fructose corn syrup is labeled as glucose-fructose, isoglucose, and glucose-fructose syrup. So why does high-fructose corn syrup have so many different names?

Because food manufacturers know you, and consumers are more aware of how bad it is for you. They are attempting to disguise that their products contain high fructose corn syrup by calling it something else. It's the same.

So, you want to break the Habit of drinking soda or diet soda because it is bad for your health and weakens your immune system.

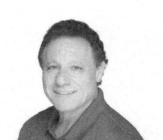

ABOUT DAVID: My name is David Medansky. People hire me to show them how to improve their eating habits to lose weight, have more energy, feel and look better, and be healthier without going on a diet; because most diets are extreme, temporary, potentially harmful, and designed to fail.

Bottom Line: You will get results without needing to buy expensive meals, supplements, or products and without having to follow a specific exercise program or count calories.

"When you eat for health, your weight loss journey will take care of itself." – David Medansky, The Health Maestro #BeTheHealthException

48

TAKE ONE DAY OFF IN THE WEEK TO RESET

DENISE MILLETT BURKHARDT

Why: Most major religions call for a day of rest, and there is a scientific reason why it works. In everyday life, we are constantly attached to our devices and online 24/7. The world is full of noise, and every now and then, we truly need to shut down and quiet the static. There are plenty of scientific reasons why taking a day off could really transform your life. Today stress levels at work are higher than they ever have been, creating havoc to our physical and emotional health. Skipping breaks can lead to exhaustion as well. Sitting all the time takes away the motivation for healthy living as well. We have to take time to move and rejuvenate. Did you know that chronic stress depletes your immune system? Weekends can provide extended R&R. When you take time out for yourself, you are also more creative. Just taking that one day off can rejuvenate your senses and give you some creative break-throughs. It might not seem like it, but by pacing yourself by taking a day off, you can be more productive during your workweek. Working more hours is not the way to be more productive. Taking a day off will help you reset and be prepared to feel motivated for your workweek. Focus on your work will improve when you take time out from work and devices. Being in the present and enjoying your surroundings or enjoying family or spouse time, or even a walk outside of your working space can lift you up and prepare you to engage more during the week. You might even find joy and passion about what you are doing if you take a day off during the week. Studies show that you're more likely to succeed in all your pursuits when you care for your physical, mental, and emotional health.

THE UN-HABIT: GLASS HALF EMPTY ATTITUDE

Why: When we talk to ourselves, we should think carefully about what we are saying. The words that we speak and the thoughts that we think are the messages we tell ourselves are true. Are you a glass half empty kind of person or a glass half full person? Studies suggest that personality traits, including optimism and pessimism, can affect areas of your health and wellbeing. The positive thinking that comes with optimism is a significant part of effective stress management. Effective stress management is associated with many health benefits. But you can learn positive thinking skills if you don't have them now.

Positive thinking does not mean you don't have bad days, and you ignore less pleasant situations. It just means that you productively approach things. You believe the best is going to happen and not the worst.

Some health benefits of positive thinking include increased life span, lower rates of depression, less distress, resistance to common colds, better cardiovascular health, and better-coping skills during hardships and stressful times. During the day, stop and think about what you have been thinking. Start small by focusing on one area to approach more positively. Be open to humor and give yourself permission to smile or laugh, especially during difficult times. When you can laugh at life, you feel less stress.

You can practice positive self-talk with one simple rule. Do not say anything to yourself that you wouldn't say to someone else. Be gentle and encourage yourself. If a negative idea comes to your mind, respond with a positive affirmation. Practice makes perfect. When you strive to be more optimistic, you will learn to handle stress differently and more constructively. You will, over time, notice a complete difference in your all around wellbeing.

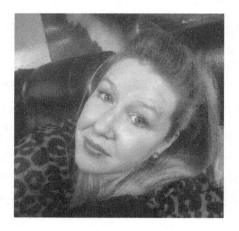

About Denise: Take a day off and reset your life. Be kind to yourself with optimism and you will succeed.

49

THE FOUNDATION OF THREE

MARK ARETSKIN

Why: It is habitual for me to look at three foundational things requirements, functionality to deliver it, and limitations in any activities.

Almost forty years ago, when I was an engineering student. I was given a product development methodology, which helped to perfect all my creations. It is based on analyzing those three fundamentals, and it became habitual to look for them in my everyday life.

It helps determine multiple solutions for certain task resolutions, lining up those solutions such as pain scale in a doctor's office, then selecting the best development path. It helps to discover the most important problems to deal with and find the best practical solution. I even got an award from one of the companies I'd worked for saying, "He knows where the problem is."

This methodology helps one reach the best results quickly without searching for shortcuts and loopholes using the traditional methods.

As an example, let's take a look at the everyday task of food preparation.

Let's imagine that we are making a beautiful and tasty cake. We will need certain ingredients like flour, water, eggs, sugar, etc., these are our requirements. Our functionality is how the ingredients react between themselves with or without adding heat to form a dough with the required viscosity and density. All Ingredients are placed in a special form (cake pan), so the finished cake will look presentable; these are the limitations.

I described the analysis of those three fundamentals in my book Invention Factory Blueprint, available on Amazon for Kindle. It's written from the inventor's point of view, but these fundamentals are universal, and you will face it in all activities you participate in. Thomas Edison wrote that he discovered 10,000 ways how not to do things. Using this methodology helps to clarify and shorten the traditional process of trials and improvements. Use this method, and all your creations will be perfect.

THE UN-HABIT: DELAYING NECESSARY ACTIVITIES

Why: Procrastination is a habit of delaying necessary activities, and it is eating at our time to be productive.

I am not talking about a short reflection on unavoidable tasks like those necessary to calibrate your tools and instruments. I am talking about delaying starting anything, including the most necessary of actions. It is especially unwise to procrastinate if you are facing a firm deadline. Most high school and college students learned this dreadful Habit by preparing for tests and finals too late. You deprive yourself of valuable time to create and refine the deliverables. Necessary but delayed tasks take away a person's attention from other things still in the works, which is one reason for diminished quality.

On one side, procrastination is a manifestation of fear of failure; by shortening the time between start and deadline, it multiplies the chances of failure several times.

Also, It creates false fillings of business with diminished productivity. Procrastination is psychologically exhaustive, and final results are rushed because you procrastinated in starting, which is a thread to your credibility. Procrastination is a process, and delaying the result may manifest insecurity and uncertainty—there a list of methods that could be used to overcome procrastination.

Not delivering could be a source of depression based on missed certain future opportunities. The first will be dividing the project into smaller meaningful steps when the deliverable would not be overwhelming as an original one. The second would be selecting the best deliverable solution based on the analysis of the requirements, functionality, and limitations discussed above. The methodology of analyzing requirements, functionality, and limitations we discussed earlier will help break procrastination because it shows the most feasible ways to achieve desirable results in an organized fashion. Procrastination needs to be eliminated.

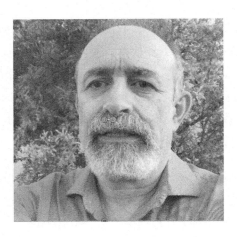

About Mark: My name is Mark Aretskin.

I am the founder of the inventors' help company Perfect Invention(R). We are part of inventors' help industry business to business oriented service company. We are helping inventors with idea development, engineering, prototyping, and referrals. Our book Invention Factory Blueprint is available on Amazon. We would like to help our customers even more.

50

SCHEDULE SOMETHING EVERYDAY
ANGEL TUCCY

Why: When the world shut down, like every other speaker on the planet, every one of my speaking events was canceled. Over the next 6 weeks, 60+ live events were canceled or put on hold. Doubt, questions, and confusion were becoming the reigning posts on social media, in text messages, and on phone calls. Yet, I felt a strong calling to show up for others. I had been traveling with a team of speakers, and I felt like they were counting on me to lead the way and provide answers, or at the very least, a small amount of hope.

The first day I started receiving cancelation notices, I received a phone call from a very panic-stricken client. She was a new client who was just launching her speaking career, booking speaking events, and publishing her first book. Before she was able to create any momentum, the speaking world closed upon her.

Instead of freaking out with her, we came up with a solution. In less than 10 days, we created our first virtual summit with 28 speakers and over 1,000 attendees. The virtual summit created a result that we had never seen from a live event – over 1,000 registered guests with less than a week of promotion. Over 28 speakers from all over the country, even internationally, we're able to participate without leaving their homes. Solutions show up when you do.

Hosting a 2-day event created the reminder that all was not lost, yet, it wasn't enough to sustain momentum. It would have been so easy to crawl into bed and sleep until noon every day since there was nowhere to go. Instead, I scheduled a phone call or an appointment that required me to be dressed and on-camera every morning. The daily morning appointment forced me to be disciplined, to create a habit of showing up every day. On days when I didn't feel like showing up, it didn't matter. I showed up anyway.

The daily habit turned into a Morning TV Show, broadcasting live every weekday morning, interviewing clients and other speakers who were essentially in the same boat. The Angel & Tina Morning Show allowed me to fall back to my roots in radio broadcasting. More importantly, it gave me a reason to show up every day. The habit of scheduling something to show up for every day has established an incredible Habit of discipline that has served me well.

HABIT

The Un-Habit: No more one-sies

Why: You've likely heard the statistics that less than 6% of small businesses ever make more than $100,000 a year in revenue. Hitting the six-figure mark is a milestone that most entrepreneurs set as one of their first revenue goals, yet most never achieve it. The reason most entrepreneurs struggle to make it is because we were taught to build our business one-to-one. One prospect at a time. One discovery call at a time, one client at a time. Building a one-to-one business keeps entrepreneurs busy but broke. Repeat after me, "No more one-sies." Instead, scale your business to grow quickly by building it one-to-many.

It's hard to give up a one-to-one model because it's most comfortable to have one-on-one conversations. Yet, it means you're repeating the same information over and over again, but only to benefit one person at a time. Let me encourage you - you don't have time to share your brilliance with only one person at a time. Your brilliance is being wasted when you share all your wisdom and education with only one person.

Tips to give up One-sies:

• No unscheduled phone calls. Schedule your time with qualified leads or paying clients.

• Schedule weekly group calls to answer the top questions your prospects have and to pre-qualify your leads.

• Document and record your on-boarding process – sending videos or checklists to answer frequently asked questions.

• Publish a book that serves as the answer to anyone who wants to "pick your brain".

Building a scalable one-to-many business is the only way to hit 7 figures: the million-dollar mark. When you set your revenue goal to hit $1,000,000, you'll open more doors of opportunity. Your impact on the world is even greater. When your business makes money, you can provide more goodness in the world. You can support a team. You can provide for your family. You can donate to your favorite causes. You can truly make an even greater impact when you scale one-to-many.

Look at how you spend your day. Compare it to the goals you have set for yourself. Do your habits line up? Creating daily habits support your audacious goals.

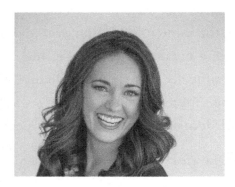

About Angel: Angel Tuccy is an Award-Winning Speaker, Radio Host, TV Producer, Best Selling Author & PR Media Specialist. Her clients have been featured on 1000's of major media publications, television, radio, podcasts, magazines, and stages.

Angel was awarded "Most Influential Woman of The Year" & "Best Morning Talk Show". She's been featured on the cover of magazines, shares stages with top influencers. She hosts a daily morning talk show syndicated on 7 streaming channels.

Angel is a best-selling author of 12 published books. Her top-selling book "ABC's of Exposure" is the how-to example for creating media exposure in less than 90 days. She shares some of the best ideas she learned from hosting over 2,500 broadcasts and interviewing over 5,000 guests. Angel has interviewed people such as Sharon Lechter, Michael Gerber, Les Brown, Forbes Riley, and Bill Walsh. Her unique approach to media is why her clients call her the Media Matchmaker.

51

TOUCH AND RESPECT NATURE

LORRIE J SCOTT

Why: The Covid Era, the era of isolation, with lock-downs, quarantines, confinement, frustration, and angst. The separation and disruption of all things important; life routines, careers, connection with elderly parents, friends, and family. The interruption of social culture; no concerts, no sporting events, no happy hours. Overnight, it's all digital; home-schooling, remote workplaces, zooms. Or No Jobs, No haircuts at ALL.

Now it is time to reconnect. Now is the time to step up our responsibility for nature instead of being at war with it. We have been instilled for the past year to wipe out the "Evil Covid Virus." Clean and sanitize your environment. Besides being isolated from other humans, we have been isolated from the natural world. A conscious effort to be active in, do for, respect Nature is important now because we are nature. To daily engage in the essence of nature immediately reconnects you to the whole of life. This connection is life itself.

The benefit of getting your hands in the soil calms the entire nervous system by increasing serotonin. Walking barefoot on the ground can restore sleep patterns. The value and merits of Deep breathing is common knowledge but easily forgotten. Sitting under a tree, smelling a rose, exposes you to healthy microbes that support your immune system. A moment of Full Sunlight on your face usually brings along with it a smile and Vitamin D. These are some of the personal benefits. On the larger scale, to step up to your personal stewardship of the planet, the climate, your food source is now paramount and will expand your life beyond the constructs of the Covid world.

These are just some of the reasons why a daily dose of nature can improve your psyche, your soul, along with literally improving and lengthening your life span and health. I challenge you to look at your world with eyes wide open to the cornucopia of life waiting to be touched by you.

THE UN-HABIT: NO RESPECT OR CONTACT WITH THE NATURAL WORLD.

Why: There has been an overall cultural indoctrination that we are alone, separate from the whole, from each other, from the earth. It didn't have to be that way, but somehow another layer of politicizing, of fear-mongering, polarities: masks/anti masks, etc., too many to list. Them VS. Us mentality. The separation set-up construct that has been amped up and beaten into us on every front. This has been going on much longer than the past year. Whether you have jumped in headfirst into the polarities or you tried to be a silent witness, your Un-Habit is to break free of the conflicts and get back to "Nature."

What if we look at this from the perspective of Mother Earth. We thought Covid was tough on us individually, but what if one looks through the sight and feelings of the loving earth:

Mother Earth's Quote:

"Forgive me, as my tears flow and the oceans rise. I don't seem to be able to stop the weeping as my soul grows heavily; yes, the physical pollution: the staleness of the air, the foulness of the water, the mountains of debris, my cherished birds falling from the sky is burdensome. The physical pain is one thing, however, the emotional agony of feeling you, my most beloved creatures, humans, tearing at each other throats, throwing hate, despair, separation, over what, nothing. I am sorry to say, it is now close to the end of this human chapter. I cannot stop my weeping. I cannot stop the decline, the fires, the changes as long as your emotional poisons fill my veins, I am helpless. Help me, help you. "

"Please, hear me, Stop, Stop for only a moment a day: touch me, care for me, do one small task, support me. "

Not all will answer, but will you?

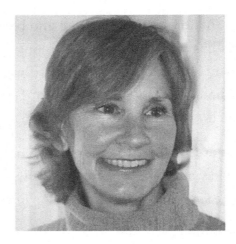

About Lorrie: In this post, Covid Era, do you want to go back to the "old normal"? Do you want to remain isolated, a slave to technology, a victim of poor habits that do not include respect and doing for nature?

Or will you choose to embrace new habits that will get you out of the box of technology and empower you to feel the pulse of life right under your fingertips? Not only the life but the magic, the empowerment of you taking action and making a difference to the outcome.

Will you choose to engage with the living or stay in the synthetic?

52

DO IT NOW

ANN KESSELMAN

Why: If you are reading this, you are at least over 1 year old, have survived covid-19, and in general made it through 2020. First, let me congratulate you for these accomplishments; my heart goes out to those who weren't as blessed and their families. This distinction allows you to implement a habit that will not only change your life but enrich it beyond imagining. It is a simple concept often scoffed at or looked at as irresponsible by some, but in my opinion, is key to a fulfilled life. It is "Do IT Now!"

How many of those that are no longer with us put off having that special bottle of wine or beautiful expensive chocolates to enjoy someday. The someday that didn't come. Didn't take the time to stop at their bucket list location because they were rushing off somewhere else with the promise of coming back someday. Meant to start putting money aside for the future to protect their family but will start someday. Put off telling their soulmate something very special that would have meant the world to them but was waiting for a special occasion someday. Their somedays will never come.

How many put off learning to play the guitar or the piano or taking a whirl at painting or hang-gliding? Or have you been meaning to get in touch with distant family and friends but put it off for later? It is easy to stop dreaming and believe that dreams are possible. But let us continue imagining ourselves experiencing luxury travel beyond our borders, roughing it backpacking in our national parks, or exploring unique primitive cultures.

We are not guaranteed tomorrow; we only have right now. Now is the time to be experienced and savored fully. These moments become memories. They should be appreciated and stored. Not to relive, since you will be living the current moment, but stored as knowledge, skill, expertise, and understanding to draw upon to make the current moment the best experience possible.

By opening yourself up to what is happening in your life right now, by daring to dream daring to be and act differently than those with limiting vision, by realizing your life deserves your passion and not putting off your" IT," you are giving yourself many precious gifts, not the least of which is never having to say, "if only".

THE UN-HABIT: NO, WON'T TRY IT. I DON'T LIKE IT!

WHY: Ok, this one drives me nuts: *"Nope, I won't try it, I don't like it!"* which quickly elicits from me a frustrated *"BUT YOU HAVEN'T TRIED IT to tell if you don't like it"*

This is one habit that needs to be obliterated, purged, smashed, erased, smooshed, eliminated, deleted, expunged, annihilated, in fact removed from vocabulary forevermore!

Ok, I get it, you get wicked heartburn, and you don't want to try that Spicy Sriracha dish; I'm not talking about that. You get a pass because that is a physical restriction.

But everyone else, I'm talking about new experiences that open you up to inspirational encounters and opportunities you would never have access to without bold exploration. A simple example is that I have a friend who would never even try beets; it took him decades until he finally gave in and tried those purple round things. To this day, he regrets 30 years of missed eating what has become his favorite vegetable.

When you don't step up and take control by doing what is unfamiliar or uncomfortable, you rob yourself of life, enhancing experiences, and the opportunity to grow. I'll often hear, *"but I don't know how, and I might fail."* My reply is *"great fail,"* that is a wonderful gift from taking bold action. Your failure just shows you one way that something doesn't work, Hurray that's a success; you now know what doesn't work, so you may work at the next possible solution.

Today, we have available many coaches and mentors who have already gone through some of these experiences so we can take a short-cut and mirror their success. The optimum word is mirror, that takes action, that takes you stepping up and risking the unknown, picking up that 2,000-pound phone, or tasting those odd-looking purple round things on the table.

You may still not like it, but you will have had the experience to draw your own conclusions and truly know it is not for you. Perfect example, I have a friend who went skydiving on his 60th birthday because his wife really wanted to try it. He wanted to do "something different" to celebrate this milestone birthday. It wasn't something he really was interested in doing, but he decided the experience itself outweighed his trepidation. She loved it, and he loved that he did it because, after that, he knew he never wanted to do it again—knowledge through experience.

It's the habit of not trying in the first place. When you are not willing to at least take the risk to do something you've not done before, that is the Habit that needs to be eliminated from your lifestyle.

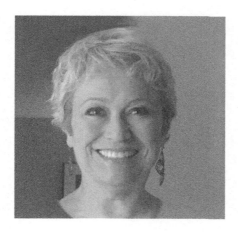

About Ann: I am the Dream Achiever. Beyond being a survivor of losing my life partner of 42 years and defeating a rare cancer myself, I've become a THRIVER. I'm the Chief Troublemaker and co-founder of my life-embracing business AMK Global Enterprises where I help you dream again, find your path to making your own dreams come true so you can escape the ordinary and live an extraordinary life!

Your Lifestyle goals are my business focus—your desire to enjoy life through exceptional travel experiences is what I provide (at wholesale pricing.)

Let's fill your *Inspiration Treasure Chest* with exciting and influential travel experiences, with an inside-out nutritional solution that supports your health and vigor. With skin luxuriously elevated by minerals from the lowest point on earth, all orchestrated to help you successfully live the Lifestyle of your dreams.

53

A YEAR IN THE MAKING

ASHLEY ARMSTRONG

Why: When you live abroad internationally, you quickly make new friends and lose them just as fast as an ex-pat. Over 14 years, I've helped hundreds of new ex-pats settle-in, create businesses, find jobs, learn the language, the customs, as well as helping them pack up and leave just as fast. Due to a lost job, can't find work, can't pay rent, no money to move back to their home country, sell everything in order to leave... that's the reality in many cases. The transition story was always the same: Hard, harder, and the hardest experience of one's life.

When you transition from a life once lived "this way" and then all of a sudden, you need to pivot and learn to live life "another way", it can feel like a 1000 pounds of pressure. Honestly, from personal experience, it's more like 2000 pounds of pressure. One of the hardest experiences in my life was moving my home and family back, starting all over again, and looking for work.

Luckily I was gifted with the knowledge of "HOW LONG IT WOULD TAKE" to feel settled again, which made all the difference in the world!

Here's Why: As a Canadian living in Cabo San Lucas, Mexico, the lifestyle was amazing, but it was 50 years behind, like the wild-wild-west. All rules go out the window, new rules get made up on the spot, and there is nothing you can do about it. You have to be adventurous and resilient because there is no income or tourism stability. For such a beautiful place, being a top destination in the world, it teaches you a lot of hard lessons on how to transition fast!

Here's How: Know in your gut that the only thing you can count on in life is change! Even if you are prepared, be ready to get thrown a curveball, so do your best to roll with it. Be OK with the fact that it's going to take at least a year or more to get back on your feet. You are not alone; a lot of people experience this length of a transition period

Reinvent yourself and thrive in a post-COVID world by not expecting answers immediately, knowing it will be a YEAR IN THE MAKING!

The Un-Habit: Inability to see your own sand timer

Why: Do you know how long you will live? If you did know, do you think you would change how you are living your life?

Why is it that many of us live life as if it's nothing special, as if you are in a video game and have 3 extra lives if you die? Why do we hold ourselves back, or why do we think we can't make the change we are yearning to make? Apply for a new job, move to that city, start that business, eat that cake, go ask that person out?

On the flip side, why is it when people who have a near-death experience "TRANSFORM"? They re-prioritize what's important to them, they slow down and just live a fuller life. It's like they are a whole new person, and they don't have time for anyone's bullcrap. What can we learn from those who have seen the pearly gates, you might ask?

Well, apparently, the average person lives 27,375 days! Yes, you read that right, you can google it.

To bring some perspective to your life, I want you to calculate how many days you have been alive thus far. You can google that too.

I've been alive for 14,196 days (38 years old as of Feb 12, 1982)

Now take the average number and minus the days you have been alive!

27,375 - 14,196

My calculations tell me I only have 13,179 days left of my life (on average). Meaning, I am past my halfway mark! If that doesn't scare you straight, I don't know what will?

Ask yourself, if you NOW see a possible endpoint, does it change the way you will live your life moving forward?

Think back on your years; how many days do you remember? Wouldn't you agree that most days pass you by unnoticed?

We tend to only remember days when something big happens when we create an unconscious anchor in our life by something amazing or traumatic. Most of our life is on autopilot. Our life's story becomes non-perceptible or discernible in the mind.

Think about all the experiences you "put off" or "saved for later?" Do you want to live with regrets? Everything can change with just one choice, sparked by one conversation in one moment.

So, I will ask you again. Do you know how long you will live? If you did know, do you think you would change the way you live your life?

Reinvent yourself and thrive in a post-COVID world by paying attention to YOUR SAND TIMER!

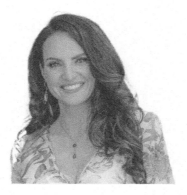

ABOUT ASHLEY: ASHLEY ARMSTRONG' The Hidden Rules Expert' founder of an eCommerce consulting firm specializing in helping product companies find millions of dollars they are leaving on the table, through eCommerce and leveraging the power of Amazon. Nominated for The Best Amazon Consultant by SellerPoll 2020 and featured in Entrepreneur, Business Insider, Thrive Global, CBS, NBC, ABC, and FOX. Her exclusive 3-step system helps private clients and members discover unseen revenue without additional inventory investment by properly positioning their product lines in order to build a loyal customer base and increase sales an average of 140% in 30 days. Think of Ashley Armstrong as your eCommerce 'Hidden Rules Expert' to take your business to the next level.

54

SELF-CARE IS A CONSCIOUS MINDFUL CHOICE

JENNIFER MORRIS

Why: Be the "self-carer chief" every day and live a 100% conscious life in mindful choices. This Habit of being your own 'Self Carer in Chief (SCIC) will change your life, emotions, and health. An SCIC is someone who gets clear about their needs and wants and empowers themselves to live and create from this information, thereby loving themselves and others better. Honoring myself in every choice as a caring partner and embracing my best interests! I live in conscious, mindful choice. The Formula for staying in CONSCIOUS MINDFUL CHOICE, as an SCIC first, care about myself, then check in with me - what do I want? Does my body say yes or no or later or maybe? Second, validate and honor this knowledge -and then third, actualize this caring LIVE IT! Immediately release backlash- guilt, and shoulds.

Celebrate me! This is my conscious (I clear out the clutter of other's opinions and my 'shoulds') mindful (I pay attention to my body, heart, soul, and mind) choice (I decide!) In all of us, this knowledge lives! Once upon a time- at age 30, I had a great job opportunity in deep southwest, rustic, rural Florida. It was good pay, challenging work, provided a promotion. My friends said, "take it, it's a perfect job." They got a lot of me right... yes, perfect job... but they did not know, deep inside of me, my hate for hot, rural places goes much deeper than the average complainer. First coercive, well-intentioned friends pushed the 'yes 'then the "should- er" showed up. (We had a long history.) I took the job...but there was wet heat, it was lonely, and the culture was rustic, there were no stores, but there were bugs, and finally I quit/got fired. (Misery effects job performance). If I had been a SCIC I would have checked in with my body "–NO!", It would have screamed, "we don't do rural wet heat rustic!!" I would have then cleaned out others 'desires "for" me and my own "shoulds". Then my clear "YES!" would have been CRYSTAL CLEAR NO - My actual Truth. I would have had some mild remorse- ok, a "perfect" job isn't there every day, BUT... guilt, fears, and 'shoulds 'would not have owned me. Fast forward 30 years later, I am now a hard fought SCIC. I release the guilt and the 'shoulds ' and stand solid in my TRUTH - living in two cities!! Listening to my 'Self carer in chief ' clarifying how to love me! This is my conscious (I clear out the clutter of others and my own 'shoulds') mindful(I pay attention to my body, heart, soul, and mind) choice (I decide!)

THE UN-HABIT: NO TO UNDESERVED (NEUROTIC) GUILT

WHY: Neurotic guilt is the experience of the "guilt" feeling undeserved. For example, when one does not eat all of their vegetables and a little voice repeats, you are responsible for child hunger in Africa, and the act of stuffing your already full stomach will save African children from this hunger. The dilemma- to walk away from the table leaves you with the difficult feeling of guilt. To relieve the guilt, you stuff yourself. But.... wait a minute? You're feeling stuffed, powerless, and GUILTY, and African children are still hurting. To illustrate the difference between neurotic guilt and healthy guilty, we take the example of a bank robber. This act might be considered guilt appropriate. We might even encourage those remorseful feelings. This guilt could help, it would be rehabilitating, and the guilt could guide you to refrain from bank robbing. This type of guilt has benefits, individually and societally. See the difference?

Neurotic harmful guilt.

Today, my friend wants me to hike. I am tired and busy with an exciting work project. I say no to my friend...and. Choose my project. Before my offense against "neurotic guilt," I would have hiked and worked on the project. In fact, I would have stayed up <u>until 2 AM</u> to accommodate both demands. I could not tolerate believing another person felt disappointment or rejection. I was the "superhero" responsible for another's feelings. Real or imagined. Guilt kept me in this prison. I lost sleep, became fatigued, and had hair falling out. I lost touch with what I even wanted. I gradually hit bottom, sick, and depressed. My new unHabit was born out of this bottom, and now a big" NO" to neurotic guilt is my daily practice. I now sleep, have hair, and usually know exactly what I want. I check in with myself to discern whether my guilt is deserving or neurotic, helpful, or a hindrance. Most often, it is neurotic and a hindrance-Then I say No. I visualize a big red stop sign and a loud NOOOOOOOOO! Today, I have more friends as I have broken enslavement to their feelings. I purposefully stop eating when I am full. I do give to charities that try to save people from hunger. And every day, I choose NO to neurotic guilt, and so will you!!

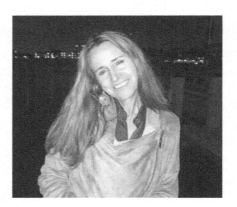

Jennifer: Jennifer Morris created The Heart of Healing, a transformational psychotherapy practice that alchemizes challenging personal histories into growth opportunities.

Jennifer moves trauma and shame into self-love and acceptance, embracing authenticity and all parts of one's self! Jennifer provides virtual psychotherapy for those in Maryland, Florida, and Oklahoma!

55

MAKE OUT AND HUG DAILY

TRACEY STARR

Why: MAKING OUT with your romantic partner or HUGGING a loved one daily is incredibly important to maintaining a heart-to-heart connection and lifelong bond with that person, plus it's great for your overall wellbeing.

"Making out" refers to a more escalated session of physical intimacy than the average kiss. Also known as groping, petting, necking, or kissing with sexual prowess.

When you commit to making out DAILY (not necessarily sex), you will find that your relationship strengthens. Your communications are more authentic and empathetic, and you feel like you are a team taking on the world together. Other life stresses tend to bounce off you both instead of taking them out on each other. This is especially important for couples with children.

And this is true with hugs and platonic relationships, as well.

Spending just 2 minutes a day in physical union not only feels amazing, but it leads to more physical contact, which is good for the body, mind, and spirit connection within yourself and your loved one. Holding hands, cuddling, and skin-to-skin touch are also wonderful ways to connect, as well.

BODY - Making Out and Hugs both release serotonin, dopamine, endorphins, and oxytocin, which promotes trust and bonding, building a special connection that furthers social development and intimacy. They also reduce the steroidal hormone cortisol. These physical acts strengthen the immune and endocrine systems, reduce stress and anxiety, headaches, insomnia, balance the nervous system, and support good cardiovascular health. Some claim it also slows aging and helps control appetite.

MIND - Physical connection helps us mentally and emotionally get through painful or stressful situations, lower depression, alleviate existential fears, promote good feelings, motivation, self-esteem, self-confidence, and a strong sense of love, protection, security, strength, and support.

SPIRIT - Embracing loved ones conveys many thoughts and emotions without saying a word. Melting energies into One gives a sense of oneness with a loved one, as well as the Universe. It's an energetic bath and spiritual connection that is beyond just the body and mind. These bring peace, tranquility and calms the soul on a higher level.

Overall, daily displays of affection, touch, and attention improve the quality and wellness of life.

Making out and hugs is a great habit, to begin with as they cost you nothing, make life easier to manage, and give you more positive results with yourself and your relationships than you can imagine.

Do yourself a favor, make it a habit to make out with your partner and/or give someone you care about a hug TODAY! It benefits you both!

The Un-Habit: Stop Toxic Self-Talk

Why: Toxic self-talk has harmful effects on your body, mind, and spirit. It creates disease in the body, mental illness in the mind, and promotes doubt over faith.

Essentially, it's a dream killer, which, if left to fester, can cause you to wonder if life is even worth living.

You are not alone. We all have an inner critic. Generally, we are harder on ourselves than anyone else.

Sometimes this little voice helps keep you safe, motivated, and reminds you of great memories or projects a happy future. Your inner critic may prompt you to choose a salad over the cake or exercise rather than escaping into tv or social media.

However, this voice can also be harmful and destructive, causing excessive negative thinking and a physiological and emotional downward spiral. This can create significant stress,

324 | 1 HABIT TO THRIVE IN A POST COVID WORLD

not only to you but also to those around you, which can negatively impact your relationships and life. It also makes you terribly unattractive and repels others, or worse, attracts negative people and undesirable experiences.

Common negative self-talk statements start with "I am not...", then fill in the blank. "I am" are the most powerful two words in our Universe. You are claiming you are that... happy or not happy, healthy or not healthy, wealthy or not wealthy, worthy or not worthy, etc.

Negative self-talk is an inner dialogue you have with yourself that limits your ability to believe in yourself and your own abilities and to reach your potential.

Lack of self-love, self-confidence, self-esteem, or self-worth can cause depression and anxiety, which block you from living your best life.

Negative self-talk also stops you from taking action towards your goals, as you cannot see your value nor the opportunities the world gifts you.

Click the switch! Consciously monitor your thoughts. When you notice your negative self-talk statements arise, switch them, and make them positive. Instead of "I hate...", try "This is challenging, and I prefer...". Be gentle with yourself, but mute the negativity when you catch it.

Focus on the good in your life, with gratitude being the greatest of all feelings for creating the life you desire. Focus on who you want to be, rather than who you don't.

Create a vision of your future. Set goals, surround yourself with positive environments, situations, and people will help you shift toward positive self-talk so you can find and live your passions, be successful and fulfilled, and live the life you dream of.

Be the best version of yourself now and break the habit of negative self-talk!

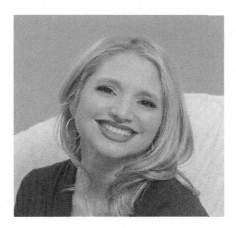

About Tracey: Tracey Starr, formerly Tracey Samlow, is the Heart 2 Heart Connector™, renowned for making heartfelt, authentic connections with people and providing introductions that lead to success and make an impact personally and professionally.

My goal is to be of service, helping you find and connect with people and resources that positively impact your life and business so you can be the best version of yourself now and live the life you desire.

56

FIND YOUR ANCHOR DAILY TO LIVE IN FLOW STATE

MICHELE DRAKE

Why: Reflect on a time in your life that you felt supported, excited, blessed, and happy. This is a state we can train our brains to move into on a regular basis. The more consistently we pattern the ability to reach these high-frequency sensations, the easier it is for our brain to arrange and revert to it—literally a habit of appreciation and gratitude. I like to refer to it as a FLOW STATE.

The neurons in our brains are triggered by a connection to a pattern that has been repeated over the days and years - just like when we exercise and want to improve our strength, we need to have patience. The steady and persistent effort can rewire the "go-to" emotions to learn the art of responding rather than reacting and to flipping a downward spiral vortex to go the other way. Energy and mood are powerful, and we can harness this to our favor ourselves and those that we affect.

This is NOT due to circumstances beyond our control; the state is definitely IN our control. When imposed tactics of restriction are in place, it is up to us to recognize our happiness as a choice and find an anchor to remind us to respond rather than react. Focus on what you want and what you can control rather than the opposing options. Some anchors that I have in use are:

1. Press the tip of the tongue on the roof of your mouth

2. Using your thumb to tap that hand's fingertips

3. Deep breaths with a hold or suspension at the top (if no hypertension present).

So it goes like this, something triggers you in a not-so-desirable way, and you, in turn, recall and perform an anchor that links you to the sensation of Flow State. A friend taught me to state Cancel Delete - every time a negativity arises inwardly. The more habitual, the more joyful you will live.

If you are having a hard time recalling these emotions or feel you have never felt euphoric before, you can try being of service to others. It is in this place of giving energy to others; you may witness how it raises their vibration and, in turn, will be a gift to yourself.

The Un-Habit: Move out of living in fear.

Why: Fear lowers our immune system "Psychologists in the field of "psychoneuroimmunology" have shown that state of mind affects one's state of health." The saying "Worried sick" is entirely legitimate. Some of us are genetically wired to be "worriers," others are "warriors." Just as mentioned in the habit above - rewiring of the brain is in our control. You are putting yourself at undue risk if you ignore the message here. Chronic Anxiety suppresses the immune system and increases our risk of infection. "Anxiety about the unknown (such as our risk of COVID-19) can hyperactivate the fear center in the brain called the amygdala. This is one of the oldest parts of the brain in the study of evolution, and it operates on a quite primitive level.

Our stress system is triggered for high alert, and both the mind and body are affected. It remains in this Fight, Flight or Freeze response as long as we are feeling anxious. "Research shows that the mere suggestion of danger, even if it never is experienced, is enough to trigger the amygdala and activate the stress response." This is one of the reasons people stay awake at night, lying in bed, worrying. It also suppresses all the beneficial functions of our body from working well as the parasympathetic system cannot work optimally or sometimes at all when the stress responses are triggered. Therefore digestion, assimilation of nutrients, repair of muscles and organs, etc., along with damaging our cells and upsets many body functions.

What can we do to improve this circumstance that befalls our everyday existence at the moment? Ancient tried and true, simple, low to no cost relaxation techniques. This includes but is not limited to

1. Breathing exercises - the body can't feel as it is in fight or flight if you are breathing 4-6 breaths a minute. It flips the switch to parasympathetic, where all rapid healing happens.

2. Meditation - this is not elusive; with a habit, you will find the way to alter states.

3. Relaxing bath

4. Relaxing music and rest.

Living out of Fear and Anchoring into Flow State and LIFE is AWESOME

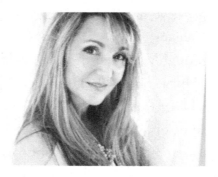

About Michele: Michele Drake - Age Reversal specialist - started an online coaching platform with 30 years of expertise as a fitness & alternative health mentor

Working with executives, entrepreneurs, leaders, and their teams who want a strategic, holistic, and structured approach to health & well-being that encompasses every aspect of their work, life, and ergonomics of their day.

We deliver a program called "Master Habits," which focuses on 8 pillars of wellness to enhance a positive outlook and mindset.

Together, we build resilience and peak performance while reducing overwhelm and stress, increasing vitality and energy, while enhancing productivity and relationships.

The expert support system allows participants to experience compounded results leading to sustainable and impactful change.

57

PREPARE AND PROTECT YOURSELF
MYLINDA BEACH

Why: When this pandemic started, I realized I was an "Essential Worker." I would be in a vulnerable position, and I had a choice to give up my job and stay home in fear or choose to remain in the job. I decided to learn about the virus and do everything I could to prevent getting it while working. My position is 99.8% office work.

I rely on public transit to travel; therefore, additional protection was required. The first thing I did is learn the latest available information and keep up with the new knowledge. Knowledge acquired included public transport precautions, which fortunately was allowed to run for folks like me. Also, what type of masks and other wearable devices I could use to lower my chances of contracting the disease.

Most government guidelines we have to help people prevent the spread of the illness to other people but not as much how to avoid getting it. The hope is if you have a medical condition that the virus can take advantage of, you will stay home. If you live by yourself, it is not so easy to avoid going out. When NYS was in PAUSE, I still had to go to the supermarket to shop as most stores did not and still do not allow someone on food stamp programs to pay for food and delivery. The one program in a trial pilot for this is Amazon Fresh/Pantry, which does both; provided you have internet to order and purchase the items via their site.

The virus doesn't do well in moving air, so taking a walk while it's a windy day is an excellent way to get outdoor exercise. Choosing alternate public transit options when they are too crowded to be protective, even with mask policy, is another right way to limit exposure. I do budget now to accommodate rides via Uber/Lyft as I know I only have to consider the driver, and they are required to disinfect after each ride. I wear neck gaiters when I'm walking in the open area or working within my office area; I do use and recommend the blue masks you can buy anywhere or a washable valveless mask that allows the N95/KN95 inserts. I wear these masks under the gaiter while ensuring they fit correctly, making sure air can't escape around the nose, and fog up my glasses. If your glasses fog, you do not have full protection.

The Un-Habit: Avoid living in fear

Why: If you look at any news site, you know that their best control tool is to create compound fear. It is avoidable. If you live in fear, your body lives in a fight or flight state, and prolonged exposure to this is horrible for one's health. The stress hormone cortisol wreaks havoc on the brain, and if you also happen to suffer a mental illness, its toll is even worse. While you are in this mode, you lose the ability to think critically or logically. Your only concern is how to survive whatever perceived problem is threatening you.

In this pandemic, people have chosen one of two paths to deal with this issue. Deny or accept. Denying helps no one, and these people end up being the main spreaders of the disease. They do not protect themselves or other people and live as if there is no problem. Those who accept that there is a virus do their research. They prepare as best as possible to keep themselves from getting it and prevent others from catching it if you happen to be one of the asymptomatic carriers.

Doing things like avoiding face to face meetings with friends and family, getting both vaccine doses, and getting delivery of goods and foods are all things you can do that can help with limiting exposure.

These actions are not living in fear; they are smart ways to go forward. If you need to host a multi-person gathering, making sure people are covid tested and safe before the event is also an excellent idea. Guests will not be as fearful of going, and you are doing as best you can to limit the chances of exposure.

Using platforms like Zoom also are excellent options and allow people that wouldn't be able to make it due to distance also to attend.

Knowledge and preparation are our best options for going forward. As long as we are willing to do our part, everyone will be cared for, and we as a whole will recover from this faster, and the next challenge will not be as challenging!

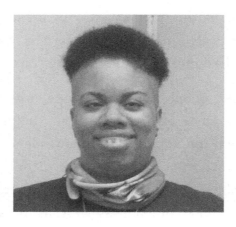

About Mylinda: Currently designing and creating an all-age coloring book and has an upcoming 50+ page positive words coloring book. These are perfect companions to unwind with after a long day on Zoom.

Mylinda has written several short stories and is slated to publish a webcomic based on humorous true stories taken from the workplace.

We all need a little humor, and life is colorful, so let's enjoy it.

58

CREATE YOUR OWN DREAM
DK WARINNER

Why: When is the last time you thought about your Dream?

How long has it been since you took time to Dream? What would you dream of achieving if you were completely free?

COVID-19 showed us something very, very profound:

We cannot rely on our routines.

Think back to the past week, the past month, that you have lived. How much of that time was intentionally directed? How much was simply resigned to carry out your routines, however valuable those routines may have seemed? How do those routines differ from the ones you were using before COVID?

We have moved past the point of no return - the world will not return to the routines that supported us before.

It's time to move to the next level - Creation!

Where we don't live the life, someone else created for us, or passed on to us from someone else, or designed by another to benefit them, not you.

What is your Dream?

If you haven't spent much time dreaming lately, take a moment for yourself right now, and simply reflect until the dreams you were considering before come back to mind.

Is your Dream right to pursue?

Does it benefit you while helping others? Does its realization add value to make the world a better place? Does it right a few of the wrongs done in the past?

That's good.

What can you do, right now, to move forward toward the realization of your Dream?

Find your way to your Dream realized, and set some milestones along the route. What do those accomplishments look like? What would you need from others to reach those points?

Write all of this down. Clarify the vision of your Dream realized until you can see the picture with razor-sharp clarity.

Then, with your Dream in mind, continue creating!

Not so long from now, you will begin to see results - results that align with your Dream. Stay on course!

By the way, when most of our natural routines are disrupted, there's a lot more time available to create - no more excuses. Get going!

THE UN-HABIT: AVOID NEGATIVE NEWS

Why: Before COVID-19, I never would have believed that watching the same news, over and over again, would have a cumulative impact on my sense of well-being, my energy, and my ability to move forward to deliver value confidently. The news was progressively depressing! For weeks after the shutdown began, my colleagues and I were basically shut down emotionally. No business was coming in. Every ten minutes, it seemed conditions were getting worse. When would we be able to return to normal?

Having lived with COVID-19 at our doorstep for nearly a year by some counts, it is clear that we are not returning to "normal" anytime soon.

So, there's no point in watching the news to find out when!

Turn it off.

Get some fresh air outside, instead!

Meet with a friend by video conference (ZOOM(R) or similar).

Plan a virtual workshop.

Catch up on your writing backlog. Remember, all of those articles you wish you had "back then"? Write them now, and they'll be ready to submit at the push of a button.

Finish up a larger project you've pushed out.

Virtually visit your extended family, especially the relatives you're out of touch with.

Oh, and that daunting list of 1200 leads you haven't started reaching out to? How about reaching out to 5 of them today?

By reclaiming the time you were spending keeping up with every repeated current development (at least, the ones they wanted you to know about), and by reclaiming the FOCUS you had before COVID-19 came on the scene:

You stay on track, and potentially even accelerate.

You also become much more resistant to being manipulated by the media's version of "public opinion". Better able to think your own thoughts in the idleness of a calm, collected mind.

That sounds almost peaceful, doesn't it? Not to mention more productive.

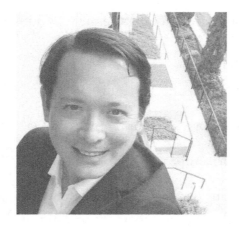

About DK Warinner: He suffered an accident at only age 2 that left him with serious chronic anxiety - after turning that around, he helps corporate professionals and others eliminate their anxiety, stress, and overwhelm, taking them from Stressed to more Successful than potentially ever before.

DK Warinner is the author of 3 books on Marketing, Customer and Client Retention, and Stress Elimination, a mentor of more than 100 professionals, host of the Center of Calmness podcast, and has been chosen to represent companies like Navistar, FMC, and Harsco.

He loves empowering others to Acknowledge the stress that holds them back, Activate their own mind-body mastery, and Achieve potentially more success than ever before – literally saving his students a 10+ year learning curve.

59

MASK UP YOUR TECHNOLOGY
NICOLE SCHEFFLER

W hy: To thrive is to do more than just survive. The 2020 pandemic created a global wave of change and accelerated digitization. It changed how companies are collaborating while adjusting the supply chain in real-time. Simultaneously, we've had to abruptly step up our relationship with technology in all aspects of life in this brave 'new' world. More virtual work and people were connected than ever as we experienced this together as one world.

As a result, more things are connected than ever before. Practical security should now be a basic Habit for everyone. Here are five simple security steps to make it a Habit:

1. Know the Basics

It's more important than ever to have secure passwords. Try using a sentence like "I Love Technology" and use the letters ILt with numbers and symbols for a password. Turn on two-factor authentication. Also, do not use the same password for your main email accounts as you do for other sites. Consider a password saving application, such as 1Password or LastPass. Things like this are a place to start, but reach out for basic security advice.

2. Own your data

Know where your data lives and have redundancy. If you get a ransomware attack and the attacker posts a number to call, take a picture of the screen with your phone and immediately power down and disconnect from the Internet. Then, contact an organization like fraudsupport.org.

3. Layered Security

Security for the network, cloud, and endpoints. Think of all the places that attacks can enter and secure them.

4. Consider the Source

Be careful with links in emails and messages and always think twice before you click. It's easy to do a quick check before clicking on the link. Just scroll over the URL before clicking.

5. Have a backup plan

Know how to restore your data. Get a solar-powered charger so you can charge your phones in an emergency.

Technology provides a way to do everything these days, and it will continue to be key in solving problems at home and in business. Keeping these five simple steps in mind is part of the movement of universal technology acceptance. Companies and individuals must accept these Habits to protect themselves in a borderless world. We had to take extra precautions against the COVID-19 virus, and our technology lives require the same protection. We must come together to protect from computer viruses and threats in the same way. So grab your digital mask, and let's stay safe on the Internet.

THE UN-HABIT: DON'T LET TECHNOLOGY MANAGE YOU

Why: Do we control technology, or does technology control us? Now that we are living behind a screen from the safety of our homes, our relationship with technology has changed. Video technology has accelerated to connect millions of people across the world, and there is no shortage of content to consume. Traditionally, we use technology and the Internet to enrich our lives, but it has become a necessity during the pandemic. We have become exponentially more dependent on technology.

While technology services us, we must make sure that we are leveraging it in positive ways that help us achieve our goals. We need to learn to master technologies for all of the good it offers, but be careful not to let it overtake our lives or prevent us from being present. Ask yourself, "Is this use of technology serving my goals?"

Here are some ways we can shift away from the Habit of letting technology manage us:

- Avoid taking your phone to bed with you.
- Manage screen time and stick to your limits.

- Put the phones and screens away during meals to connect with others.
- Diversify where you source your information to get a well-rounded picture.
- Balance the negative news coming into your life with more positive content.
- Start the day with your own meditations, vision, and affirmations instead of immediately opening social media. Let your first thought of the day be focused and intentional.
- Look for meaningful online friendships/communities with people you have things in common with that can help your mental state during the quarantine.
- Consume information related to your goals.

When we are more aware of how technology impacts our lives, we can see how important it is to manage our relationship with it. Don't let it prevent you from showing up in the world as your authentic self. Stay true to who you are. People want to see the real you, even if it is behind the camera. Ultimately, we must be the ones managing how we consume technology in our new world and be aware of what it brings into and takes out of our lives. When we manage the technology we need, we can unlock its benefits while remaining grounded. Like all things, our love for technology is best with some boundaries.

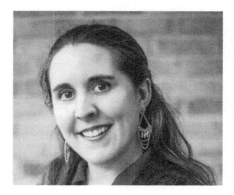

ABOUT NICOLE: Nicole Scheffler is a Tech Diva dedicated to sparking success for women in technology careers – women who are working to own their career success and realize the impact in a male-dominated field. Nicole empowers women with proven success principles to define their aspirations and goals and boost their daily contributions in the digital world. In a fast-paced technology career of more than 16 years' Nicole shares her wisdom in her best-selling "Pillars of Success" book with Jack Canfield. With hundreds of hours interviewing women in tech on her podcasts, Nicole's experience provides a clear success framework for women in all stages of their tech careers. Her courses, content, and speaking help tech divas fires burn brighter.

60

WRITE WHAT YOU WANT DAILY
HEATHER RINE

Why: This Habit is vital to implement into your life every day because it will shift your neuro pathways. Not only will you begin to believe what you're writing, but also start to open yourself up to the changes that need to happen for you to reach your goals.

For example: have you ever felt frustrated because you haven't been able to break the ceiling on a particular income goal? Have you begun to notice that you have an increasingly limited mindset because Covid is affecting your income? You may be able to generate your ideal income for a brief time, only to find yourself sinking back down into an income status that just isn't serving you or your family. You're not alone.

What causes these recurring results are learned thought patterns, cultural stigmas, and socioeconomic class that we inherit through intergenerational transference. These lessons are taught to us from infancy and middle childhood and can contribute to the limited beliefs in what we *think* we can earn and what we actually bring home.

The incredible thing is, though, many of these beliefs and Habits we are holding onto aren't even ours. We inherited these neuropathways from various external experiences, where ultimately our subconscious plays out programmed responses that contribute to our success, or lack of it.

My mentor, Bob Proctor, teaches us that a proper self-image is key to getting what you want. If you want to live the life you desire and earn your ideal income, there has to be an alignment with your self-image through thought patterns.

Imagine your life as a movie where you're in charge of the script. This is incredibly powerful because how you see yourself is how the rest of the world will also see you. Let that sink in.

Would you think of your best friend, spouse, or children the way you think about yourself? No? Then it's time to change your self-image. The same applies to people you are looking to work with. If you don't believe you're worthy of the money you're asking for, why would anyone else? How can a supervisor see your worth if your self-image is poor and projecting the energy of lack?

This is where it's essential for you to write your own script. You need to see yourself as worthy. You need to see yourself as someone who people can't wait to give their money to, because if you're just hoping that someone will see something in you that you don't, then you're giving over your power. And when you do that, you are stealing away from your greatness.

This process is incredibly powerful because once you've identified the belief you want to shift, we just need to create a new Habit to correct the mind. Yes, changing a simple Habit in how you view yourself will significantly contribute to creating a life you love and can't wait to wake up to each day.

THE UN-HABIT: INCOME LIMITING BELIEFS

Why: When you come from a place of lack and believe that you can't earn any more than you already are, then you are experiencing a belief that has been passed down to you intergenerationally. These beliefs are our autopilot. For example; we get up and automatically go into our morning rituals, no conscious thinking required. Maybe you shuffle to the kitchen and grab a cup of coffee, automatically thinking about how you don't feel like dealing with your boss, or you don't want to deal with the bullshit at work that you don't get paid enough to endure. Then you wrap up the getting ready for work ritual, drive or commute to start your day while still thinking cynical, lack less thoughts. Sounds fun, right? Sure there are some good times and amazing folks we get to experience during the day, but does that deposit of pay reflect the value you bring?

Changing this waking up Habit, writing your new thoughts until they become your new autopilot is the key to changing your life. You're engaged in changing the emotional connection from a lack, to an abundance mindset that writing new thoughts creates limitless pathways.

When I played softball, I was a solid player, and I maintained my position as a starter for over ten years. There were a few intimidating pitchers throughout my career, so when I knew we were playing against these teams, I had to really focus and not let fear screw up my batting game.

My catching game was always on point because I always had a winner's mindset and a lot of confidence when catching. When I played, I batted in the fourth position (if you don't know baseball or softball, this is known as the clean-up batter, so the team counted on me, not to strikeout). I needed to bat everyone around the bases. Once in a while, I would walk up, take my home run stance, and hit a couple of foul balls. When this happened, it would start to shake my confidence, especially if the catcher was talking shit and the pitcher had that grin that said they knew that it would be easy to defeat me. I knew that I had to snap out of it so I would step out of the batter's box and repeat to myself while I took some intimating swings, "you're the clean-up batter, you're the best batter on the team, you've got two on base that you want to bring home, you're amazing and have this in the bag." And without fail, I would get that hit, those cheers, the butt smacks and hugs and admiration from my coach and teammates.

But what if my thinking went the other way? Well, many times it did, much like the Habit with money. If we allow our Habits to play out and don't disrupt non-productive thought patterns, we don't learn. If we don't disrupt those patterns, our behaviors will never change, and we will never receive the results that we desire.

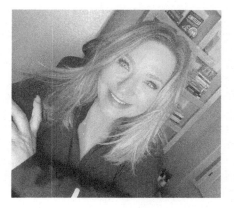

About Heather: My clients prosper through my Thinking Into Results mentoring, which guides them through the process of tapping into their limitless potential using cutting edge mindset innovation.

61

LEVEL UP & IMPROVE THE SKILLS EVERY DAY

FRED MOSKOWITZ

Why: Has there been a skill that you have always desired to learn, such as speaking a foreign language, playing a musical instrument, storytelling, website design, or social media marketing? What about public speaking, networking, sales techniques, or negotiation skills? Perhaps you have been thinking about taking up standup comedy, real estate investing, fly fishing, classic French cooking, or gymnastics. Pause for a brief moment to think about something that you have always wanted to learn more about. It can be practically anything at all, such as technical skills, business skills, soft skills, or even hobbies. The available resources are endless, and it does not matter your age, profession, or level of experience. All it takes is for you to set the intention and then follow through with the drive and desire.

The post-covid world affords us endless opportunities to develop our skills and expertise with education and training, which are now widely available through online learning platforms. In today's modern times, we are afforded unique opportunities to learn new skills and technologies, and all it takes is for us to embrace the new medium of online learning. A cursory internet search will turn up endless options for you to explore - master classes, workshops, tutorials, and educational training programs. Seek out and connect with the top masters and influencers in the areas of expertise that you are seeking to grow, and participate in sharing knowledge that is taking place.

Modern technology and social media make it so easy to seek out and connect with the top performers in just about every field. This is an amazing opportunity that we simply cannot pass up. Visualize in your mind how enriched your life has become or how your business will have grown due to those new skills that you can begin to build today.

I would like to share this famous quote from one of the world's most influential mentors, Jim Rohn. He taught us that "Formal education will make you a living; self-education will make you a fortune."

In this post-covid world, it is more important than ever to dedicate time and resources to our self-education. Lean in to this concept and get started today!

HABIT

THE UN-HABIT: BREAK THE HABIT OF RESISTING CHANGE

WHY: Instead of resisting change, consider the benefits that can come from embracing change.

The world is filled with people who have been comfortable with the way things were done, people who benefit from things staying the way they are, people who, by their general nature, are resistant to change.

They may fear a loss of status or a threat to job security in their organization. They may have a vested interest such as financial gain or status, which would be lost or impacted by the change.

Academic research has shown that humans are hardwired to resist change. The brain's natural response is to interpret change as a threat. It will respond with a physiological reaction known as the fight-or-flight response, triggering adrenaline release into the body.

When life hands us change, think about the way that we can respond. Many people will be sitting idle, just waiting, and asking when things will get back to the way they were. Instead, we can use the opportunity to innovate, pivot, and come up with new methods and ideas that can propel us forward in the world.

Find ways where we can bring value to the marketplace. We can be asking our clients and others around us what they need and then come up with a way to provide that to them. Instead of waiting for things to change back to the way they were, we can be the ones to effect new and innovative ideas and concepts.

When we embrace change, we take a moment to ask ourselves, "How can I show up in the world with a new and innovative idea, product, or strategy?" We show up ready to take some risks, test out some new ideas, and bring new concepts to the marketplace. In return, the world begins to see how we are showing up as a leader, innovator, and forward thinker.

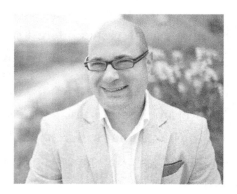

About Fred: My name is Fred Moskowitz, and I'm known as the alternative investment guy. Why alternative investments, you may ask? Well, growing up, I saw people around me make all kinds of foolish financial decisions that set them up to fail and fall behind on their goals. If they only knew about better options, they could have succeeded and not been taken advantage of financially. There are better and different ways; my mission is to share these alternatives resulting in a positive impact on your finances. My clients have dialed into my financial strategies using the power of alternative investments to create passive income streams. Do your ears perk up when you hear these words? You can learn to diversify outside of Wall Street. Become knowledgeable about investment strategies intangible assets like real estate and mortgage notes; you'll learn how new opportunities become your alternative income strategies!

62

PRACTICE FORGIVENESS DAILY
EMILIO ROMAN

Why: Forgiveness is a practice that has saved my life. Without understanding the true meaning and reasons to forgive, I was living a lie. On the outside, I had portrayed that all was well, but inside I was corroding with anger and resentment. Illness and pain overcame me to the point I wanted to end my life. I began to internalize this energy (Anger & Resentment), and it nearly destroyed everything I cared about in life to include my children and relationships. My military career also took a hit, and I ended up in rehabs and court-martial type infractions in my beloved Marine Corps. Alcohol and Drugs became my friends, they would not leave or punish me, or so my warped mindset had me believing. I had buried multiple childhood sexual abuse by uncles to the point I believe they were just dreams I was experiencing. But my body knew, and it was communicating to me to release this life trauma. I felt shame and guilt and questioned my sexuality.

I was in a bad place. Thankfully, I was re-introduced to Forgiveness but not from a religious perspective. Meaning, Forgiveness was a Gift I was giving myself to release the hurt that kept me in active addiction for so many years. Also, I learned Ho'oponopono (The Ancient Hawaiian Art of Healing & Forgiveness). Four Key phrases (more like mantras) one says when you desire to send love and light to an individual who has wronged you or you have wronged them with your words, thoughts, or deeds. I am sorry; please forgive me; thank You, I love you. While these words are not new to anyone, when they are strung together with this powerful intention of releasing blocked energy, nothing short of miracles happen immediately. The shift is so real; family and friends who know you for years will notice you talk, walk, and even look different. A load has been lifted which weighed you down as you moved through life. This is the Power of Forgiveness at work.

THE UN-HABIT: I WILL NEVER FORGIVE YOU

Why: The Habit of holding on to petty feelings or justified resentments will kill you slowly. It has been said, "Resentment is like taking poison and expecting the other person to die."

If you have ever had someone hurt or harm you physically or emotionally, you understand, thoughts of getting even or seeing the other person pay for what they did to you are very typical.

The fact is this, hurt people hurt people. If we have never been taught a process of how to forgive or release this low energy will not serve you, there will be a build-up of emotions. Ultimately, happiness and fulfillment will seem to allude you.

You will create an unconscious Habit of becoming sarcastic and even attract people, places, and things that vibrate on this low energy.

I know this firsthand; I was that guy that wanted to argue the finer points of politics and religion given the opportunity.

I never walked away feeling good about myself for the simple reason, if I felt I won the verbal jujitsu, that meant there had to be a loser, and no one wants to be a loser or made a fool.

Even when I made the case or argument, the energy never felt right. I even lost friends or those that could have developed into lifetime friendships.

This unforgiving attitude of mind will bring into existence ill health, which will affect your mind, body, and spirit 100% of the time without fail, its universal law.

Today, I believe science is catching up with ancient wisdom from the Bible, Recovery Institutions, and practices like the Hawaiian Ho'oponopono (The Ancient Art of Healing & Forgiveness). Saying the serenity prayer out loud or in silence will immediately begin to shift your mind's vibrational force and add new life energy into your current situation.

"God grant me the serenity to accept the things I cannot change, the courage to change the things I can, and the wisdom to know the difference'"

The Ho'oponopon practices use four powerful simple yet powerful phrases, I am sorry, Please forgive me, thank you, and I love you. Whatever your religious or spiritual flavor, you would have to agree, these four expressions are heartwarming to the soul in any language.

Letting go is the opportunity to experience this journey we call life more fully and abundantly.

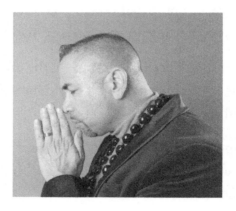

About Emilio: Celebrity Fitness Expert Emilio Roman has excelled in the health and fitness industry for over 20 years. His zest for fitness began at the age of 12, and since then, he has spent much of his life dedicated to helping people reach their fitness goals across the nation.

Tapping into his warm, friendly personality, Emilio is a master of fitness motivation and possesses a rare combination of fitness knowledge and inviting communications skills to help anyone change their perspective on fitness.

A native of Camden, New Jersey, Emilio joined the United States Marine Corps to further his passion to be challenged and to serve his country. He served four years of active duty (plus four years inactive) in the Marines, where he earned a reputation for training top military officials. After his time in the Corps, Emilio followed his passion for fitness by becoming a certified personal trainer and establishing himself as an elite trainer at major gyms and fitness centers on the east and west coasts. He has trained celebrities including Queen Noor of Jordan, as well as professional athletes with the Toronto Blue Jays, and the Houston Astros.

Today, Emilio is focused on bringing his core message of Spiritual Fitness (Gratitude, Forgiveness, and Service)to schools, Universities, and Faith-Based Organizations around the world.

63

LOOK FOR THE PEOPLE WHO WILL ELEVATE YOU

TERESA CUNDIFF

Why: I will confess that I wasn't on the lookout for people to elevated me when 2020 began, but God was! He brought Forbes Riley into my life through a friend, and my life has been transformed forever! Through Forbes, I met Charles Vest, Steve Samblis, Sara Pugh, Sherri Leopold, and so many others. Through those people, I have met Greg Reid, Shannon Parsons, Brian Smith, Scott Duffy, Angela Totman (Sharon Lechter's Assistant), Jen Du Plessis, Maresa Friedman, and I hope to meet so many more this year! Through other introductions, I now am connected with powerful women I look up to named Keri White and Elizabeth Valdez, who add value to my life. A man named Kyle Helm is also a "go to" guy for me. Name dropping aside, the most important thing you can do is to start making connections! Positioning yourself now is key to being ready for a post COVID world.

There is no need for you to feel alone and flounder. Another critical decision I made in 2020 that changed everything was taking a course that reinforced what I already knew I was great at! Proofreading!! I am a credentialed proofreader because I stepped up and took a really hard course that many people can't pass! I challenge you to seek out what you're good at and what you love doing. It took me a lot of 2020 to nail down that I love grammar, punctuation, and sentence structure and that I'm really good at finding errors in written work. It's second nature to me. And it took mentors to help me cut through all the "noise" if you will and hone in on that...but once I did, so many things began to click for me. Connections are key. John Donne's famous quote, "No man is an island" is as true today as it ever was. If you don't have mentors, you must seek them out.

We have especially learned through quarantine how much we need interaction, thank goodness for the internet, and seeing people over Zoom and Skype. Find a person who excels in your field and connect with him or her. You want to emulate a person who has already leveled up in what you want to do. If he has a Facebook group, join it! If she has a business page, of course, like it, and go to notifications for that page and set it to receive all of them, not just the highlights. If you feel "stuck", a mentor will help you push past what is holding you back! Intentionally surround yourself with people who are where you want to be, who bring a positive mindset to work and have a good word for you.

You have value, and you bring value now and always! Know that and embrace it! Set yourself up for success in a post

COVID world by aligning yourself with mentors now. This book is filled with them. Smart mentors have mentors themselves!

The Un-Habit: Let go of Habits that no longer serve you

Why: If you have ever let others define you, it's time to stop that! That is a terrible Habit of which you may not even be cognizant, and it's time to make 2021 the year where you heighten your awareness of that fact and remove things from your life that no longer serve you. It's time to remove things that no longer contribute to you leveling up in your business, in your health, in your personal life, and your overall mindset!

Please understand that I am preaching to the choir because I certainly don't have it all figured out! I am a work in progress and look forward to reading what the other contributors say here. But in a post-COVID world, we all need to come to grips with the fact that the "old normal" will never return! It's just not going to happen. A paradigm shift has occurred, and we all are given the same opportunity to "reinvent" ourselves. I use that word for lack of a better term. We've all experienced a shared trauma with this pandemic, and everyone has his or her story to tell. What do you want your story to be for 2021? I want mine to be one of growth and triumph! One where I finished the book I've started; one where I've helped anyone who reached out to me; one where I found success in numerous ways that's not just measured in dollars. How am I going to do that? The same way we all can - to remove from my life the things that no longer serve me or contribute to my growth as I move forward into 2021 and life after COVID.

You will have to determine for yourself what those things are. Still, this chapter is here to bring to your awareness that you need to make connections with great people to level up just like me. You also need to remove Habits, possessions, places, and sometimes people (yes, people) to level up. But sometimes it's just that you are lazy. Or maybe, you should just make better choices about where you're spending your time. Just take stock, I guess, is what I'm really saying. Do a deep dive inventory of all aspects of your life and look for where efficiency is needed. It's what I'm doing, which is why it's the forefront of my mind.

I kept the last New Year's resolution I ever made, which was to never make another New Year's resolution. You see, I give myself permission to start over every single day if that's what I need. It's called grace. Take stock, but also give yourself grace! It takes a lot of courage to make bold moves, and it's going to be scary! I just have to love myself enough and remind myself that I matter. YOU matter too! Pivoting in a post-COVID world requires moves, but the groundwork needs to be laid now, and you need to make yourself a priority!

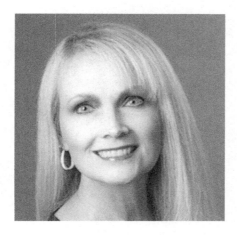

ABOUT TERESA: Teresa is a credentialed freelance proofreader who makes her clients' writing shine! Her tag line is, "I know where the commas go!" And she certainly does. Her credits include "Ninja Sales Secrets" by Charles Vest. Her love of words has sparked in her the creation of a Facebook community called Wordy Nerds Academy. Each day of the month, she introduces a new word with each letter of the alphabet to increase the Wordy Nerds Nation's vocabulary. If you have a writing project that needs an extra set of eyes, reach out to Teresa. She is here to help.

64

ALWAYS KEEP YOUR OPTIONS OPEN
BLANEY TEAL

Why: So you are probably thinking about how is "keeping your options open" a habit... well, throughout our lives, we are trained to say "NO." Ultimately, our subconscious brain is there to protect us, thus; resisting change or alternate ways to do something. So that means you may be closed off to opportunities that could change your life. What if you had said NO to that first date. Or what if you said NO to the job interview. What if you said NO to change all the time. NO is easy.... No is a decision. But what if you said NO at the wrong time.

My dad gave me some great advice as a child. "Always listen to every opportunity, you can always say NO" This advice has served me well over the years. In these post-covid times, you may be presented with opportunities for a job or a different way to do something that you have done a certain way for years. Your first instinct is to say NO right away. You may even feel some angst in your body physically. This is resistance. But instead of saying NO, try listening to what that person has to say. Even go as far as to sleep on it before answering. It's OK to say, "let me sleep on it, and I'll get back to you tomorrow." Thanks to my dad's advice, my life has taken many amazing turns, and I have had incredible experiences that I would have missed if I said NO without listening first. So always keep your options open.... when someone gives you advice... listen... when someone wants to share something exciting with you...listen... then sleep on it and circle back with them... and it's OK to say NO. Still, you may find yourself... thinking YES! This habit will keep you from missing out on something that could change your life forever!

THE UN-HABIT: NEGATIVE THOUGHTS OUT TO THE UNIVERSE

Why: So I am a true believer of what you think about, you bring about. You've probably heard of "The Secret," well, I'm here to tell you that the power of your thoughts are real!

It's so easy to wallow in negative thoughts. And even worse, to say them out loud. Be VERY careful what you put out to the universe...If you say you can't pay your bills, you WILL get more bills.

So here's a little trick I learned a long time ago. When you slip and say something negative, immediately. SAY OUT LOUD "Cancel, Cancel, Cancel" and reword your thought.... I know it sounds hokey, but I promise if you catch yourself and fix it right away, you will start to change your habit of saying negative thoughts. I mean, who wants to walk around all day saying "Cancel, Cancel, Cancel," it could get very tiresome. You are reprogramming your thoughts. So instead of saying I don't have enough money to pay your bills. Start by saying, "Money flows easily and effortlessly to me from places known and unknown, expected and unexpected." This UN-HABIT has totally changed my relationship with money during Covid and beyond.

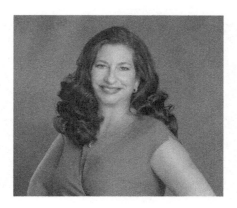

About Blaney: Blaney Teal is a mompreneur who knows how to pivot in challenging times. Blaney's passion is helping business owners create unique virtual expos, conferences, and summits online. She brings business professionals together to grow their network through her networking organization MBX: Making Business Connections. She is also the Next for Success Academy founder, helping entrepreneurs fine-tune their mindset, skillset, and toolset. Author of the upcoming book "The Lunch Date: Why Skipping Lunch is Hazardous to your Wealth."

65

SELF CARE FOR BIPOLAR DURING QUARANTINE

AMY MORRISON

W hy: Taking even a small step in your self-care can be a massive step for you by creating a positive Habit that will make a huge impact on your mental and physical health with the bonus of feeling confident through the accomplishment of taking action.

As someone who has the diagnosis of Bipolar, I learned through hard experiences of the symptoms, how not practicing self-care, took a huge toll on me even with just it being a month into the quarantine.

In April of 2020, at the beginning of the shutdown, I took action with my self-care by pivoting my mental health through exercise. It was the start of putting into action the Habit of exercise that was non-existent for years and affected my mental health negatively from not doing so.

One day I saw on Facebook that the creator of The SpinGym was going Live through Zoom (the virtual meeting rooms). I had ordered one the year before yet didn't learn how to use the exercise tool. For me to want to exercise, it must be fun. I quickly learned from the tool's creator, Forbes Riley, that it is extremely fun to use! By Forbes being one of the 1st Fitness Coaches to use Zoom for empowering people to keep exercising while at home, it also created a way for me to be connected to positive, energetic people.

Have I fallen off the new habit wagon? I sure have. It's given me another way to practice that is so important to self-care, "Grace". Remember to give yourself grace because these are unprecedented times that everyone hasn't experienced before.

THE UN-HABIT: LACK OF SELF-CARE WITH BIPOLAR

Why: Self-care for people with Bipolar is not optional. Bipolar symptoms can amplify during the quarantine. Thus taking care of ourselves is even more important than usual. As someone who has the diagnosis of Bipolar, I learned through hard experiences of the symptoms, how not practicing self-care was taking a huge toll on me even with it just being a month into the quarantine.

The infamous "Covid 15" took effect. I ate whatever I wanted, sat around extremely more than I used to, and struggled even more with exercising. All this activated my symptoms. The symptoms I get with Bipolar are anxiety, anger, rage due to the depression. All of it amplified from my Habit of not practicing self-care. I've heard so many times how exercise was an important part that helps calm the symptoms. Yet I didn't take action, which led to shaming myself for not doing it. By shaming myself, it perpetuated not taking action from beating myself up in my mind, with talking mean to myself for not doing what I knew I should do.

In not practicing the habits of self-care that relates to Bipolar, we give the disease power over our lives, instead of us using our ability to take care of ourselves by creating positive habits.

Has it been a struggle to start the Habit of taking care of yourself through exercise? From someone that too has this struggle, I encourage you to use the extra time we have during the Pandemic Quarantine to take an action step by implementing an exercise that inspires you to keep your new Habit alive and exciting for you. By creating your new Habit, it will have you feeling accomplished, create confidence, and you will inspire others to also empower themselves through self-care.

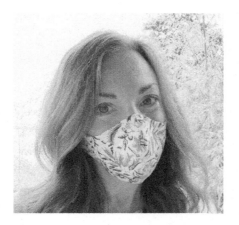

About Amy: This is some (insert the tongue out silly emoji here) Roller Skating, Ballroom Dancing, concerts with dancing & jumping involved, well dancing in general, are the fun ways for me to exercise.

I also don't want to take 30-60 min every day to exercise. That was stopping me too. Taking on the Habit of exercising by using the SpinGym, I've taken my power back from beating myself up for not doing it, and it feels so great to do what I know to do while having fun!

Are you looking for a fun, fast way to exercise and start your new 1 Habit powerfully through Self-care? I highly recommend checking out SpinGym on YouTube. It's Zoom friendly if you're sitting in a chair in meetings all day, super portable, and inexpensive, which helps for those of us struggling with finances from losing work.

Keep in your mind that you aren't alone in your self-care with bipolar! Literally, if I can take on the exercise portion of self-care, you can too! In the words of the group Snap 1990, your positive Covid affirmation is... "I've Got The Power"

66

FINDING WAYS TO CONNECT
AVA BOUDI

Why: On normal days, it's hard to count how many times we got physical contact with others. For several isolating alone, this could be the longest period in their lives that they have gone without skin contact. The intense distancing we're seeing now could be, one would hope, a temporary change. But as more countries begin to lift their lockdown measures, we are faced with the matter of the way to return to reality. How will we interact with one another in a way that keeps us safe but doesn't offend?

For months we've been practicing social distancing, keeping a minimum of two meters or 6 feet away from one another, avoiding touching communal surfaces, and stifling coughs and sneezes. It's been challenging to change a lifetime's worth of experience of societal norms that demonstrate politeness or affection: in many cultures, we recognize that how we greet new people, hug those we look after, or offer a hand, literally, to those that need it, may not be welcomed anymore.

Now that we're hopefully preparing to travel out into the globe again, all those ingrained habits may need to stop. The French's double-air-kiss beloved might be a vector of transmission; the nice and cozy embrace of an Italian greeting is potentially too dangerous. "Touchy-feely" behavior generally could cease to be acceptable, and with it, everything we've learned normally filled with physical contact might change.

For me, this social distancing is very challenging. Although I grew up shy, I used to see and meet people, network for business, and enjoy hugging my friends. I think making friends is one of my skills since once I get a friend, they usually stay around many years! I create a community for my work online for my clients of Avahosting Internet Solutions and my supportive and networking community at my online Busy Mom Magazine. But this pandemic would not stop me from doing that, and I just have to do it virtually! Which, of course, is not the same. Being a networker and connector, I love to collaborate, listen, and mingle with others, especially my loved ones. At the same time, nothing can truly replace the in-person hugs, hello's, high-fives, and happy moments. My habit saved me in this pandemic. I turned it into a positive habit that helps people in their boredom and loneliness. In turn, it helps with my boredom and loneliness. I schedule virtual visits with friends and family. And I have tools to keep in touch. I will continue to connect to others and them to each other with my Mom's TV Channel and make it interactive.

The Un-Habit: Stop living in isolation and loneliness

Why: I set up everything that I need to continue this habit. I upgraded my computer, increased bandwidth for my internet, and installed all the software that I knew may help, like zoom, skype, WhatsApp. Devices that make loved ones feel closer like Alexa is often used by people I know, and the Facebook portal. I got a green screen and a ring light. We can hang out with online services like Amazon, Netflix Party, Spotify Playlist, and Steam. Watch parties, Discord, Twitch, Amazon, and more.

Staying at home and avoiding crowds is necessary to prevent coronavirus spread, but it can lead to feelings of isolation and loneliness. Reach out. However, you can, and talk about important things in life. I'm high risk because of breathing issues, so I've hardly been out or around other people. Not even in stores. Pre-Covid, I used to love to browse stores and walk outdoors with friends and family.

I have to work extra hard as a shy person who doesn't know what to say. But we can all try. At least send a "Hello, I'm just calling to see how you are". Usually, when you call someone on the telephone, they are going to say a little more than just "Fine, thank you for asking." Let them know you really want the details!

If they can't talk or you have a hard time communicating, ask them to send photos and create your own photos at home.

Some days I just look forward to the delivery person coming to talk about the weather and wish them a good day or a good holiday. I can see the postal worker from my door, so I usually say hello from far away if I'm not too busy working.

Do what you can to reach out.

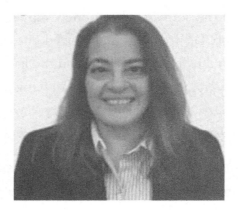

About Ava: Ava Boudi, is from NYC, New York. She started in the 1980's promoting nightclubs and managing bands in NYC building a large marketing and distribution network, she launched the careers of many popular solo and group disco and dance artists of that time and some rock bands too!

In the early 90's she was an Editor for a Humanist newspaper distributed in Chelsea, NYC, called the Chelsea Journal.

In 2007 she was among the pioneers of podcasting as a Podcast Consultant and was a regular at Podcamps and other digital media conferences. Later becoming Co-Publisher of Podcaster Whos Who Online Magazine and Co-Organizer Podcamp City Online, a online podcasting conference, long before there were online events like today.

She is also a community leader with her local community group she founded, and a county wide recycling group of almost 3,000 residents of Queens County, NY She has won awards and accolades for her community service.

Today, she is the Publisher and Managing Editor of Busy-Mom.Com Magazine, and the Moms TV Channel on most streaming services. As well as Owner of Avahosting Internet Solutions.

67

TAKE TIME TO DE-STRESS EVERY DAY
JACQUIE DOUCETTE

Why: We live in a crazy-busy world, and with pandemic worries added in, it's not going to get better anytime soon. It doesn't matter whether you're the CEO of a major company or only in charge of yourself. Every morning your brain starts making lists of the activities you have to accomplish that day.

This happens even before your feet hit the floor in the morning. Many high performers have notebooks by their beds to write down the thoughts that come to them just before they go to sleep or jot down ideas that come out of their dreams... before the thoughts are lost upon truly waking. They do this because it relieves the stress of keeping that idea in mind throughout the day. By writing it down, they release the space that it holds in their brain so something else can take its place.

When you complete a task or activity, you mentally or physically cross it off the list. But your brain doesn't really let it go. It continues to mull it over, examining what you did – and how you could (or should) have done it differently. Your brain doesn't know how to shut off on its own. If you don't give it permission to stop, it keeps turning all the time.

This is mentally EXHAUSTING! And it's going to wear you down physically if you don't get into the habit of turning off your brain for even just a few minutes each day. The longer you push yourself without giving your brain a break, the more likely you are to run into serious medical issues.

There are many ways to de-stress:

- **Meditation** – even five minutes/day to start will give your mind a break
- **Aerobic & Strengthening Exercises** – helping the blood flow through your body ensures fresh oxygen reaches your brain, clearing your mind
- **Breathing Practices** – simple wherever you are: sit up straight and breathe in deeply through your nose till your chest/lungs are full; hold for a count of five; release the air slowly through pursed lips

My favourite? Climbing into the hot tub at the end of the day and just closing my eyes for ten minutes, breathing deeply while I listen to the water bubbling. (You can do this in a bathtub too!)

I challenge you to start with just five minutes once a day. If you do this regularly, you'll see the change in no time.

The Un-Habit: Do it all, all the time

Why: We all want to be successful at what we do, right? And we're taught that success means doing "all the things." But nobody is good at everything; it's just humanly impossible.

When you try to do everything, your focus is diminished. Your brain spends time working out how to accomplish all the tasks, and the result is that each task gets less attention than it deserves. You might think you're a champion multitasker, but truth be told, you're giving each task maybe 60%...at best. And that effort isn't your best work, so you end up dissatisfied with your accomplishments, even though you've put a lot into them.

So, stop trying to do it all! Take a moment to think about what you do each day. Do you really have to be the one that does everything? Are you the ONLY ONE who can do it all? Even if you're a one-person show right now, some tasks can be outsourced... remember it's the WHO, not the HOW, that gets things done.

There will be some activities that have to be yours – as Jim Muehlhausen describes it, this is your Picasso work. You are the artist, and only you can do it properly because it's your masterpiece. But most of your daily tasks are mundane and repetitive, and you can teach others to do them. So, do that!

Once you release some of the daily tasks, you'll find that your mind is less cluttered, and your Picasso work will take less time. Your stress level will diminish, and your day will open up.

You'll find you have time for other interests; if you don't have any interests other than work, FIND SOME! You're going to have time for them now, and you don't want to waste that precious time because if you're not careful, this un-habit will come back on you. You need to close that door for good. It's not healthy to spend all your time focused on work.

I challenge you to identify ONE TASK that you repeatedly do, that someone else can take from your plate, and delegate it today.

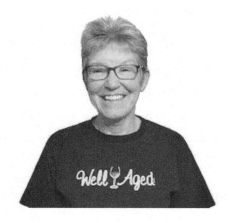

About Jacquie: Jacquie Doucette has created a community for people who know they want to retire TO something, not FROM something. On its launch, her Beyond Retirement podcast quickly hit the top charts in Entrepreneurship, Business, and

Careers, and she's routinely asked for guidance on living your best life after you leave your 9-5. Her Rocking Your Retirement intensive gives you the game plan you need to hit the road running when you decide it's time.

68

REMOVAL OF DISTRACTIONS IN OUR DAILY LIVES

MANDY MAY

W hy: We need to remember this time of the pandemic of 2020. I fear that when the virus is minimized where we can begin to live again, meaning drive a car, go to the store, see a concert, or work again, that Americans will soon forget. I fear that Americans have an innocence that they do not want to let go of. I fear political environments have politicized being safe against pathogens. This pandemic has seen families ripped apart by political views—fathers against daughters, sisters against sisters. I plan to continue to hope through conscious efforts.

I hope in the face of that fear that most Americans will continue global consciousness and remove distractions that keep us from truly living.

The changes we all made during 2020 have created a workweek that looks very different for most. There is a radio personality that I listen to that had to broadcast from home in New York. The comedy in her situation almost inevitably began right away. I laughed at her stories of kids crying on air, her yelling at kids when she thought she was muted. Her husband was walking nude in the hallway, not knowing they were on air, and colleagues commented on our current situation in quarantine work weeks. I laughed during the hell we were living in, and it helped keep sanity. Just by harnessing the Dalai Lama's sense of humor during death and tragedy, I was able to keep on keeping on. In the beginning, we all thought it incredible that just a few Americans had lost their lives. But now we are reaching beyond four-hundred thousand. It seems like many are choosing to ignore that rather than face it with hope, changes, and humor.

Remove distractions, focus on living well, and living with humor. God-willing, we will not return to the status quo. I wanted to write these points to future generations and those who might not have completely let go of our previous innocence.

• Slow down, breathe, laugh

• Enjoy your home, your pets, your kids, your partners

• Cook more, Drive less

• Talk to strangers using smiles and waves, and humor

• Seek carefree entertainment

Yes, even the Dalai Lama has had to make changes. He has debated Buddhist Philosophy with the Monastery over zoom calls, and he has made a plea to all to save our Earth from the

Global Climate Crisis, reminding us it is our only home. Specifically, we need to develop our minds and our hearts.

THE UN-HABIT: LIVING WITHOUT EXPLORING OR ADVENTURES

Why: When this pandemic began, I was teaching middle school science. March 12th, 2020. The day where everything, as we knew, began to reshape and change, if not crumble. Our world realized that a future together is much better than a future alone, or no future at all. As a teacher, I had to make an immediate pivot to creating packets and videos online for my students and parents to watch and learn. This unprecedented time called on each individual teacher to forge on their pathway to learning for all students, including those with special needs.

The aspect of being at home suddenly, with everyone under the same roof, was a bit shocking. It was a good shock, but shocking none-the-less. Suddenly being at home to help my own children with their online learning was a staggering reality that simultaneously hit the world. Flash forward to late summer, I lost my job due to low enrollment at our charter school. This was the best blessing, as we were caregivers for our beautiful mother, and we had two kids now at home. I took the new job of being the right-hand-woman to my kids seriously! It was enjoyable to be so intimately close to their learning. I was able to bring them snacks and help them with homework. We supported their technology needs. It felt good to be gaining back some time from the workweek and giving it to those I care for and love. We chose to enjoy each day.

Here is a list of how we did that; you can choose to live today too!

Things we did that we had rarely or never did before the pandemic:

• Created a campground in our backyard, complete with fire grate to cook on

• Legos, puzzles, board games, walks, workout videos

• I spoke to neighbors while on walks during the day that I had lived next to for seventeen years and never met.

• Created "Mom's Barber Shop" in my bathroom so that the kids and husband can continue to look halfway decent!

• Spent more time as a family, including cleaning!

• Cooked together as a family and baked lots of cookies

• Shopped solely online and used delivery services for groceries and other household items.

• Practiced our instruments, learned new instruments, sang, and danced.

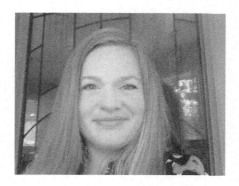

ABOUT MANDY: Mandy May has been an educator for twenty-one years. She has taught science, art, music, dance, political science, history, geography, English, writing, technology, reading, and math. Mandy is a Partner with the World Wildlife Foundation and volunteers locally to help preserve land and water for our future generations. With her insights as a mother and teacher for over two decades, Mandy continues to push the boundaries of community outreach and global consciousness by educating students on the power of humor and inquiry, allowing natural learning to occur. Mandy has had great success using this method with all students, including those with special needs.

69

FEEL YOUR FEELINGS AND EMBRACE THE PAIN

AMY GRUSSING

Why: When you feel your feelings, you embrace the pain so you can learn from it. Why do we tell our children to calm down – when the pain is there for a reason. Whether it is physical, emotional, or spiritual pain – pain gets our attention. Have you ever grabbed a kitchen pan and realized it was hot? Yes, of course, you did! Pain wakes us up and is a warning to look at and evaluate why it is there. A hot pan is easy to figure out. But what about the emotional pain you have experienced. Do you worry? Are you stressed? Do you feel anxious, especially with all the changes in this COVID-19 world? Have you ever felt butterflies in your stomach when you had to present in front of a large group of people, perform on stage, or compete in a race? How we feel emotionally affects how we feel physically.

What are we to do with our emotions when they are painful? The best habit you can start right now is to stop and embrace the emotional pain. Do this by feeling the feeling and letting your mind and body sit in it. If that means cry, then cry. Let the pain flow through you. If you feel completely sad or scared, then feel that pain and ask yourself, what is this telling me? What can I learn from it? If you are in a dangerous place or situation, do what you need to do to be safe.

As you embrace emotional pain and let the feelings emerge, you will feel a shift of energy. Sometimes it happens fast, and other times, you wonder if it will ever change and get better. But it happens in an instant. There will be a lifting, an emotional release, and your higher self will emerge. As you consider the worst thing that may or may not happen - you will remember that you can get through it! Think of the hardest time of your life, you made it through, and you learned tremendous lessons. If the pain has to do with a relationship, realize you can only control yourself: that is your actions and no one else's. This includes their opinion of you – and there is freedom when you let go and love yourself! Remember, those feelings are there to protect you and provide wisdom to know your next steps. Move forward to a healthier you. As your mind prospers, so will you in every way: body, mind, and soul!

THE UN-HABIT: DO NOT ESCAPE YOUR FEELINGS AND PAIN

Why: When you escape your feelings and pain, you find yourself turning to unhealthy habits. This causes you to be in a cycle of more pain because you get mad at yourself. Then feeling bad, the mind gets filled with negative self-talk that one would never say to a friend. An unhealthy cycle of turning to food, alcohol, drugs, shopping, gambling, porn, even excessive workouts, or any other relief - is temporary. It keeps one going on a downward spiral. You can ask yourself – how long did I feel better? It may have been 10 minutes, an hour, maybe even a day. But the feelings and pain are still there, and they become worse when we do not face them.

The solution is to stop and feel the emotional pain and evaluate it. It is ok to not be ok. When you embrace the feeling, then you can decide what to do with it. Remember, we taught our children to name their feelings. Why? Because when we name them, we acknowledge how we feel and then can respond. Is there an action you can take that will be healthier? I encourage you to write in a journal. When you write, you release your feelings. Maybe you are angry and beyond hurt by someone. Write them a letter and then rip it into 1000 pieces or shred it because you are letting the pain go! The pain is not for you to carry. When you release it, you have emotional freedom. You are getting rid of anger, rage, bitterness, and hurt.

There are many opportunities to help you through this process of not escaping your feelings and pain. Seek therapies, such as traditional talk therapy, EMDR – Eye Movement Desensitization and Reprocessing therapy, hypnotherapy, support groups, and compassionate people. Go where you feel led by peace. Take a small step; there are many people who care and want to help. One great benefit of COVID-19 is being able to connect with people that you would have never met. There are support groups on Facebook, zoom, 12 step groups like AA and Al-Anon, along with faith-based groups such as Celebrate Recovery. Find people that will encourage you and speak the truth in love. As you stop and not escape your pain, but rather acknowledge how you feel, you have taken healthy steps to a better you!

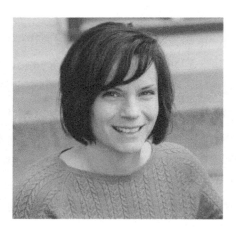

About Amy: Amy Grussing is known as The Essential Oils Stress Buster. She did not know how to manage stress - which caused her much pain in life: an autoimmune disorder, as well as physical and emotional pain. Amy persevered through these many trials - including 5 years of severe sicknesses with her son. She knew our bodies are created to heal, which put her on a quest to find natural solutions. A friend introduced her to essential oils, and her life has never been the same!

Amy learned to advocate and care for herself physically as well as emotionally and spiritually. The transformation in her, her son, and her family was so profound that she continually shares the benefits of pure therapeutic grade oils and supplements. What she loves most about what she does is seeing lives transformed, people loving and caring for themselves and living their best life.

70

BE PRESENT IN THE MOMENT
KRISTIANNE WARGO

Why: The cries are heard. The demands are made. Fill up the calendar, busyness is the way. But how does any of that bring joy and peace?

A badge of honor that clouds priorities and separates those you love from what you wish you weren't doing.

Your living legacy won't be won by how many achievements hang on your wall or all the accolades you've received in the community. The "likes" 👍 on a social media post will soon fade behind another viral video. Cats or not, you are the one who loses.

So what really matters in the big scheme of it all?

It's not what you get or what you say. The only way is presence today.

Life is worth living when you experience it to the depth of your heart. The distractions are put to rest allowing you only to see the best. Good or bad, you are there. Your presence is what's needed, not all the balls in the air.

If you could have one moment back, which would you choose? Some would gravitate towards a time where something needed to be changed for a better outcome. Others would vote for a memorable time that brought joy and love.

You see, we look for what we can control and attempt to conquer the goals from an action stance. But what is vital to today; your presence.

Chasing moments can be exhausting. Take a step back and be present. Trying to multitask and fulfill every obligation in a split second is overwhelming. Slow down your day and let your presence command attention.

What you do matters. How you choose to live your every day counts. But all will be lost if the presence is not fostered.

Presence can be achieved by taking the time to breathe and savor the moment. Breathwork makes room for all of your senses to be aware of the stimuli around you. (Source: _NCBI_) Details become more memorable and tangible.

No more, "I think." It's time to create your now!

Just because this season of COVID-19 is one you cannot control, does not mean that your life is less than. In fact, the greatest habit you can commit to is presence.

Stop playing small and commit to what really matters. With each passing moment, you have the opportunity to impact the world you touch. When you are willing to be present in the moment and observe that which you are experiencing, life becomes real.

Presence is where vulnerability blooms and authenticity grows.

Be present. Be incredible. Be YOU!!!

THE UN-HABIT: BUSYNESS RULES THE DAY

Why: Over the centuries, the advancement of technology and science has been a gift of doing more. But with that advancement comes setbacks. Your calendar soon is crammed with activities and commitments pulling you away from what was once honored as family and leisure time. Busyness rules the day.

When greeted with "How are you?", you quickly respond with "I'm so busy!" It's a badge of honor expressed proudly with your words that flow from your mouth.

But where has busyness really benefited you?

Have your relationships grown closer? Do you find the quality of time is greater? What are you gaining from not making time?

In life, there are choices to be made. Some allow others to dictate what is necessary to be successful. A mental shift then occurs, too, when everyone else is doing it. Who wants to be left out? Not me!

So busyness rules the day.

Unfortunately, though, a crash and burn season grabs your attention. Something must give, or someone will break.

Who needs to be the wonder woman and superman of the world?

Surely, you have more to offer this world than a calendar full of stuff robbing you of precious time that you can never get back. Instead of focusing on what others dictate for you, challenge yourself to look for what is necessary, what is life-giving.

Take a hard lesson from centuries ago; be willing to say NO! As the clock ticks away minutes, it's up to you to discover how to live your day.

As much as busyness seems productive, look again at what matters. Are you growing the relationships that pull at your heartstrings, the ones that give you the reason to live?

Life is precious and needs to be cherished. Whether you want to be honest or not, getting real offers a sense of confidence and opens your heart to feel more. Is being busy giving you that?

Let go of what you can't control and be specific about what you can. The busy badge of honor only excludes that which you should include.

Your presence is essential to live, love, and impact. Begin to discover what works for you and your life's goals. Don't look side to side and compare. Every day is a day to share you with the world.

Give busyness a rest and focus on being your best! Be present. Be incredible. Be YOU!

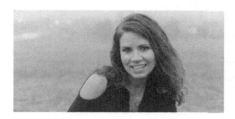

About Kristianne: I am a lifestyle strategist and executive coach who supports those who desire to love their reflection. Life is not only about the external achievements but about the internal reflections that guide the daily steps.

"One step at a time leads to miles of greatness!"

My goal is to help people become their best selves through personal development and growth and further their leadership. As the Founder and CEO of Create Your Now, the focus is driven from the keep it simple strategies, everyday solutions that conquer the daily challenges.

The daily podcast serves women (and men) in their everyday lifestyle. Topics of discussion include leadership, mindset, entrepreneurship, parenting, relationships, faith, health, and wellness.

Life is never perfect but is always lived through presence. Create your now! Take A.I.M. today with consistency and intentionality. You are called to live, love, and impact. Be present. Be incredible. Be YOU!!!

71

FIND YOUR GIFT FROM EACH MESSY MOMENT

TARYN LAAKSO

Why: Let's face the reality here; life is far from perfect. In fact, life is quite messy. I believe that 2020 illuminated this for everyone around the world. The trick to not getting sucked into the mess and letting it define you is by finding the gifts and opportunities.

Back in 2012, I thought I was in the perfect marriage. I was sitting in a big messy event that highlighted the flaws of the 'perfect life' I was living. My confidence was shattered because I was facing the challenges of divorce, being a single mom to my two daughters, and managing to live on a much smaller household budget. During this time, I started a daily habit of journaling every night right before bed, where I reflected on what I was most grateful for that day. I admit, some days were extremely difficult to find the gift in the doo-doo pile, but I was always able to find something even if it meant being grateful for waking up and surviving another day.

Today, my daily gratitude has evolved into seeing each challenge as either a gift or opportunity, allowing me to shift my perspective from negative to positive. In the past, I might have seen something as "bad" I now have the ability to see what is "good" and learn from that experience. Based on the powerful work of Positive Intelligence® by Dr. Shirzad Chamine, I can shift a negative perspective into a positive one by taking a few moments to breathe. Which stills my mind and accesses my inner wisdom to see the gifts in the challenges. This builds stronger mental muscles and neural pathways to fight off the constant inner critic thoughts permeating our brains and replacing them with positive thoughts.

One particular challenge from 2020 comes to mind. Our blended family planned a sailing trip to the San Juan Islands of Washington. Unfortunately, our electric engine had a different plan, and our trip was canceled. I could have sat with disappointment and frustration and moped around our home. Instead, I saw this as an opportunity to do some much-needed relationship building for my coaching business. That unexpected week at home resulted in four new clients filling a group coaching program that has changed the course of business in amazing ways!

As you reflect back on 2020, what gifts did you received from the challenges you faced? With 2021 upon us, spend every day reflecting on the gifts and opportunities you received from each challenge you faced. Imagine what is possible now?

HAB1T™

The Un-Habit: Inner critic rules

Why: Courage Starts With Showing Up and Letting Ourselves be Seen ~ Brene Brown

Our brains constantly fire off thoughts that keep us playing small in our life or feeling bad about who we are. For most of my life, I was constantly battling thoughts that pushed me to be as perfect as possible while believing the lie that others would love and appreciate me more if I was perfect. If I didn't feel like I could do it perfectly, then I wouldn't try it all because I might fail and look stupid. I wouldn't express my emotions when I was sad or angry. I bottled all those feelings and stuffed them deep down.

Ugh! How these negative thoughts and behaviors limited me in my professional and personal life. The kicker was that no matter how 'perfect' I thought I was, I wasn't actually happy. I was a false representation of happiness. Shiny on the outside and an empty shell on the inside. Without knowing how to feel, love, and experience life fully. I looked like I had it all together, but the essence of me inside was miserable, numb, and alone.

The road to finding my inner happiness is bumpy, exhausting, and a down and out dirty fight with my inner critic saboteurs. I am deeply grateful that I choose to intercept the negative thoughts and instead listen to my inner Sage's wisdom. The part of me that evokes empathy and curiosity within me and engages it with others around me.

You are a precipice of change; It is possible to live a life where you could let the inner critic voices become your brain's board of directors. It will get you by because its origins were a survival mechanism from childhood. You can choose to let the thought of "You need to be doing more to be successful" or "Don't bother trying if you might mess up".

Or you can decide to fire that board of directors and invite empathy, curiosity, happiness, and forgiveness into your brain space.

What type of inner board of directors do you want supporting you in your life's decisions that decide your fulfillment and happiness? It's your choice, so choose wisely.

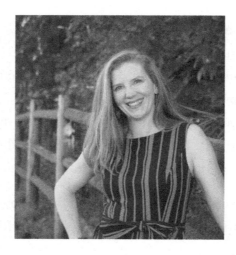

About Taryn: Taryn Laakso believes deeply in the work of Positive Intelligence® that allows herself and her clients to intercept their negative inner critic voices so that they can reach peak performance in their lives. This work has immense positive impacts on her own personal and professional life. She has taken this journey herself and has conquered personal obstacles with courage and determination, along with a fierce passion for overcoming negative self-talk. She is uniquely suited as your guide through her training as a Co-Active and Positive Intelligence Coach and her affiliation with the International Coaching Federation. She wants to help you find your strengths as a leader in your own life by empowering you with self-confidence and expand your horizons when faced with difficult challenges. Together, she'll take you to your personal summit so you can live on top of the world in your business and personal relationships!

72

APPRECIATE YOUR ACCOMPLISHMENTS
PATRICIA PEARSELL

W hy: Two years ago I had a realization that lifted such a weight from my shoulders. It was so empowering and so freeing that I began to share it with others around me. I speak this realization out loud as a daily affirmation to myself while recalling some of the things I have accomplished in my life so far: "I have accomplished much in my life, my accomplishments have meaning."

In a time that is so filled with anxiety and self-doubt making a habit of reviewing and appreciating your accomplishments on a daily basis will help you to remember all that you have learned, how you have grown, to be proud of who you are, to develop your self-confidence, and to believe in the gifts that you have to offer your families, your communities, and the world around you. I'm not just talking about reaching big goals or milestones.

There are so many events in your life, even daily ones, that when recognized as accomplishments will be empowering.

The daily practice of appreciating your accomplishments will come to be a powerful self-care tool, one that is free and already within your reach. It will show you that it is not particularly the goals or milestones you have reached, but the challenges you have faced along the way that are the true accomplishments, the gifts and the power. Every time you overcome a challenge in your life you will release self-doubt and learn to trust yourself more. For example, when faced with the opportunity to perform as a public speaker I get extremely anxious at first until I remind myself that I have been through much scarier things than talking in front of a group of strangers.

The best time of day to practice the habit of appreciating your accomplishments is as you are preparing for sleep. By appreciating the things that you did accomplish that day, rather than berating yourself for those things you "should have", you will be setting yourself into a positive mindset for a more peaceful and restful sleep, and for a new day ahead. For example, when my To Do List did not get completed, or even started that day, I make a point of recalling the events of the day. I focus on being grateful for the opportunities I had to help people that I know and love, and the lessons I learned that day. It's truly a peaceful way of settling down for sleep.

This habit will raise your vibration and attract more opportunities for growth, learning and helping others. I strongly encourage you to try this habit so that you can see how it can support your mind, body and soul. It feels amazing!

THE UN-HABIT: Stop comparing yourself with others.

Why: When you compare yourself against others it will lower your vibration and initiate a cruel cycle of negative self-talk. It may start quietly but it will eventually become louder and will cloud your ability to be grateful for all that you do have and have accomplished in your life. For example, when you compare yourself to others that are experiencing more financial freedom in their lives you will feel resentful towards them. You will also feel frustration towards yourself because you have not achieved that same financial freedom yet. You will become negative, anxious and angry and those opportunities that may help you move forward to that goal of financial freedom for yourself become more elusive. Continuing this bad habit of comparing yourself with others will lead you to the point of frustration where you just decide to give up trying and will stay in this negative self-sabotaging state of mind.

By breaking this one bad habit you will raise your vibration and you will attract more positive and personal experiences and opportunities into your life.

When we stop comparing ourselves with others we gain the ability to believe in our own lessons learned and the gifts that we have to offer. We realize that our accomplishments have meaning and value, not just for us but those around us that we love and want to help.

For example, once I stopped comparing myself with others I was able to share the knowledge and gifts that I have gained through my own challenges with greater confidence. I am grateful for the opportunities of helping others by sharing my unique story with them.

While many of us may face similar challenges in life, love, family and business, we are all individuals and truly unique. To compare our journeys step-by-step is unfair. Embrace your own journey, all of its challenges and successes. There is only one YOU and believe me when I tell you that there is value in all that YOU have learned from your own experiences. Breaking the habit of comparing yourself to others will free you and will enable you to move forward to becoming the amazing, imperfect person you were meant to be. It will allow you to truly realize and embrace the gifts you have to offer – those are your superpowers!

The only person you should be comparing yourself to is the one you were yesterday.

I challenge you to stop comparing yourself with others. Be your own cheerleader, encourage yourself and those around you and before long you will see and feel a shift in the vibrations of your mind, body and soul.

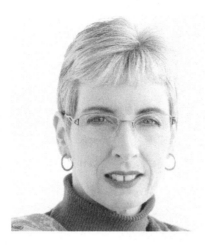

ABOUT PATRICIA: Patricia Pearsall is a Wife, Mother, Caregiver and Medical Advocate supporting family and friends as they navigate medical challenges. Having experienced her own Caregiver health challenges, she is particularly passionate about supporting Caregivers in looking after their own health and well-being. Pushing past her fear of public speaking has blossomed into many opportunities to speak at events where she has been able to encourage and support others. Over the last eight years, Patricia is proud to have helped many Caregivers and their families improve their health and wellness with whole food nutrition and nature therapy. In 2020, Patricia realized a life-long dream of becoming a published author when she was invited to become a Co-Author of 'Ignite Your Passion And Step Into Your Purpose', which quickly became an Amazon Best Seller. Being a published author has also brought many new public speaking opportunities, which she embraces fully.

73

SHUT YOUR MOUTH AND SAVE YOUR LIFE

SHEREE WERTZ

W hy: If I could instill one good habit in your life, what would it be? It would be breathing consciously through your nose.

We cannot live without breathing, and for the most part, we breathe unconsciously. It's a natural, instinctive action of our body; that we don't give much thought.

We are fortunate to have two different modes of breathing, our nose and our mouth. However, most people are unaware that we are intended to breathe through our nose. There are some exceptions, but that is another discussion.

Did you know when we are born, for the first few months, we can't breathe through our mouths. The airways of babies have not fully developed, so they don't have the reflexes to breathe through their mouth.

424 | 1 HABIT TO THRIVE IN A POST COVID WORLD

Each part of our body has a function. An obvious function of the nose is to breathe, and an obvious role of the mouth is to eat. Even though we can breathe through our mouth, *we should Not!*

We don't want to discredit mouth breathing totally. It clearly helps us out from time to time! If our nose is blocked to allergies or illness and during physical exertion, our muscles require an increased level of oxygen

Were you aware that breathing through your nose keeps air into your lungs longer than breathing through your mouth? It boosts your nitrous oxide level and provides 18% more oxygen in your bloodstream. It gives you more energy, supplies the cells with the oxygen they need to function efficiently. The highest performing athletes have breathing coaches.

The air we breathe is filtered as it passes through the nostrils. It is warmed and moistened by as much as 40 degrees before it gets to our lungs. This is particularly important in cold weather and for people with heart and lung issues. Cold air going into the lungs [from mouth breathing] can cause your lungs to close.

Our mouths are the window into our bodies. Our body is great at compensating. We assume mouth breathing is normal; the body gives us signs and symptoms that we tend to ignore. Mouth breathing can be a Habit, or it can be a sign; there is a bigger problem.

If you sleep with water next to the bed or wake up with a dry mouth, that is a good sign you are mouth breathing. You can improve your health by simply changing the way you breathe.

Are you aware if you are using your mouth, your nose, or both?

Change your habit, change your life!

THE UN-HABIT: MOUTH-BREATHING

Why: There can be some major impacts on your body when your mouth is open, based on whether you are consistently breathing through your mouth or nose.

Compared to the positive benefits of nasal breathing, mouth breathing brings on many undesirable health issues.

Breathing through your mouth tends to dry out the tissues, reducing our saliva that is supposed to wash away bacteria continually and keeps the tissue of our mouths healthy. When you mouth breathe, saliva is reduced, leaving your teeth and gums susceptible to bacteria. These harmful bacteria can kill good oral microbiome. This leads to serious conditions like gingivitis, periodontitis, receding gums, cavities, oral decay, and bad breath. Simply closing your mouth prevents bad bacteria from wreaking havoc.

In children, mouth breathing can lead to permanent skeletal deformities. Altering the position of the tongue changes the shape and growth of the jaw. Mouth breathing can result in a high palate, narrow mouth, Tongue tie, tongue thrust, gummy smile, overbite, crooked teeth, lack of sleep, and behavioral issues.

Since oxygen is our primary source of life, and exhalation is the main way to get rid of toxins from our bodies, poor breathing can contribute to a multitude of health problems, from high blood pressure to insomnia, sleep apnea, and even contribute to some forms of cancer.

Irregular breathing affects both men and women and can be a symptom one or more months before a heart attack.

Among the symptoms that predict a heart attack are insomnia, accompanied by anxiety, and low concentration. You may have difficulty falling asleep, staying asleep, often accompanied by a feeling of breathlessness or dizziness.

Chronic nasal obstruction is caused by a condition that does not go away on its own, like a deviated septum, nasal polyps, enlarged tonsils, or adenoids. It's important to see a doctor if you've suffered from mouth breathing and chronic nasal obstruction for more than a month.

Blocked nasal passages are a common cause of mouth breathing. Sinus infections, allergies, and common colds can be a temporary cause of blockages in the nose that go away after a week or so.

Generally, if you can breathe through your nose for more than one minute, it is a Habit; there are exercises you can do. Many people who start nose breathing while they sleep notice improvements in energy levels, mental clarity, and overall health after just one week.

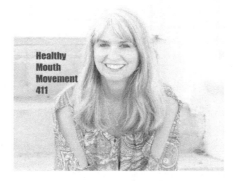

ABOUT SHEREE: There are several reasons someone might become a mouth breather. Awareness is the key to understanding. The best treatment is often prevention.

Don't be paranoid, but pay attention to your health, especially to the things your body is trying to tell you. Shortness of breath, dry mouth, hoarseness, brain fog, bad breath, waking up tired, dental and speech problems are a few symptoms you might experience.

I also offer some simple tips to help you break the habit of breathing through your mouth. Together, we will evaluate the symptoms, the possible cause(s), and what actions you can take next to live a long, happy, healthy life!

74

BE LOVE

JANICE BURT

Why: You know how they say that love and fear cannot co-exist? Well, it's true. I only know this to be true from personal experience. After the loss of my marriage, I discovered that I had been living in fear. Absolute, pitch dark, suffocating, imprisoning fear. Once I became aware of all the fear, I realized (through therapy) that I needed to replace the fear with something else. Fear doesn't just magically go away on its own to sulk in the corner. No, fear is aggressive and plays for high stakes. Fear doesn't go down without a fight. What was I to replace fear with? The answer came from deep within me. It came from that deep, mysterious place of spirit. The answer was love. I must replace the fear with love, and the love would expand and grow within me so much so that the fear would be forced out. And it worked! The more I focused on embodying pure love, the less space I had available for the fear.

Suddenly, I wasn't trapped by the fear. Suddenly, I was free. I began doing things that I had previously thought were impossible. Like running a marathon, self-publishing a book, speaking on stages, acting in short films, and competing in a bodybuilding competition. The fear no longer had control over me. It is amazing the things we can accomplish and the people we can become when we remind ourselves that we are love and begin to operate from that place. In my case, love started growing, and I was becoming more and more the highest version of myself. It may sound cliché, but love will always win.

Sometimes we get so caught up in the external world and the never-ending to-do lists and our own limiting beliefs that we forget to access our deeper purpose. Our deeper purpose is to BE love. Fear prevents us from doing this. Your life will change dramatically if you come from a place of love daily (it's a choice and a conscious decision) and allow the love to take over your entire being. Fear will be pushed out, and you will be truly content, peaceful, and more powerful than you can imagine.

THE UN-HABIT: LIVING FROM A PLACE OF FEAR

Why: Fear is the destroyer of dreams. It is the handcuffs that keep us bound and the prison bars that prevent us from going anywhere. Fear can feel absolutely debilitating. To get past fear, we must face the fear. There is no way around, underneath, or above it. The only way is through. If it sounds daunting, it is. We must take a huge leap of faith into the abyss of the unknown when walking through our fears. But this I know...it will ALWAYS be worth it.

When I was a child, I loved to talk. My dad even nicknamed me "Chatterbox" growing up. So naturally, in high school, I joined the Speech & Debate Team. I started competing in these speech contests and started winning. I was 16 years old and feeling pretty empowered. Then, halfway through my speech, I forgot my lines during the finals of one of the competitions. I will never forget the piercing silence that filled the room and the expectant faces in the audience. I lost that speech contest, and because of that one event, I didn't speak publicly again for another 20 years. That is how powerful fear is. I allowed fear to silence me. Finally, 20 years later, I did start speaking again. Sometimes, when I would stand up to speak, my body would noticeably shake. It was the fear showing up again. I couldn't hide it from the audience, so I would just stand there and shake because I knew that nothing was worse than going back into that prison of fear.

Fear will make you feel safe in your comfortable prison of familiarity, but it will deprive you of the life you are meant to live. It will strip you of a full, vibrant, adventurous, passionate, exciting, purposeful, and meaningful life. Fear is meant to keep you safe from lions and bears, but not from living your best life. When you feel, fear telling you to play small or not to show up at all, breathe deeply, remember who you truly are, look fear directly in the eye, and face it head-on. Do that thing that scares you the most. It will be hard at first, but after some practice, it does get easier. You realize that you don't die and that the world still spins and life continues on, even if you fail or look like a fool or get criticized or whatever happens that you most fear.

Your best life and your purpose lie just beyond on the other side of your greatest fear.

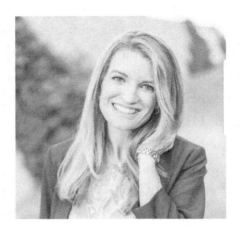

About Janice: Janice Burt aka Spanish Janice is a communications specialist. She is a Spanish interpreter, voiceover artist, yoga instructor, author, and inspirational speaker. She dabbles in acting and bodybuilding and has made it her life's mission to become the highest version of herself possible and serve others along the way. Subconsciously, she was full of fear until her divorce at the age of 37. As she became aware of the fear that resided within her, she began a gradual transformation. She went from fear to love, from dark to light, from anxiety to presence. It is a daily choice for her to stay grounded, loving, peaceful, authentic, and happy.

75

EMBRACE YOUR UNIQUE VALUE
HELEN HARWOOD SNELL

Why: The one thing that holds most people back from growing their business, career, and personal relationships is not understanding their value. We all have an individual story that makes our value proposition different (and better!) than anyone else's. Imposter syndrome is the internal dialogue we hold in our own court that deems us a fraud. It holds us back and, worse, also deprives the world of receiving what we have to offer. The sooner we can embrace our own story, the better positioned we will be to serve the world.

The great thing about stories is they never quite have to be over. There are always sequels, prequels, and even re-writes. Your story is the journey of you. It's a celebration of where you have been that sums up the value of who you are right now. Your education, personal and work experience, success, failures, grief, joy, personal relations, and talents and gifts are like no one else's. This makes what you offer to the world truly special. And your journey continues today, tomorrow, next year, and decades from now. That story will be different than it is today. But, today will always be a part of your story of who you are.

We fall prey to second-guessing ourselves and identifying our short-comings too often. The hero's journey is a classic storytelling style reflected in most books, movies, and even business content. No hero is without his/her flaws. They need a guide. They need to overcome conflict. And they need to overcome themselves, most often, to fulfill their destiny. Think of the biblical heroes God chose to highlight: tax collectors, prostitutes, greedy children. Tell me the name of any character from a movie or novel that doesn't have a flaw. They stepped into their purpose when they owned their truth. Let this be you. Be your own hero and live life broken.

THE UN-HABIT: SECOND-GUESSING YOURSELF

Why: "Say yes - then figure out how to do it later." Sir Richard Branson

There would be many who disagree with this statement. I would have been one of them years ago, but I warmly embrace this concept now with one caveat. Say "yes" only when it is in alignment with who you are. Opportunities come to us every day. The choice of friends, a partner, a college, a field of study, job, location, and business opportunities align when you follow your intuition and your natural talents.

This helps to negate second-guessing yourself because you are acting with a defined purpose in alignment with your values. When you are in alignment and second-guess yourself, you are then dealing with other factors like fear and self-doubt. Excitement shows up in your body and feels the same way as fear. It's easy to assess it as fear and back away. But what if you let the idea linger that you're excited? That's where I say, "Just do it."

Think of the quarantine, lockdown, and other emergency measures that threw businesses off course in 2020/21. There are still some waiting for it to "get back to normal". But some threw their hat in the ring and declared they would take their business online, or build globally, or start a new business model altogether. Those are the people you want to be. There will not be a return to the way things were. There never is an exact same day, or same feeling, or same customer. One of the joys of life we need to embrace is change. Change makes room for creativity and excitement. One of the worst things a business can face is routine. Customers, websites, social media, and strategic partners need to be attracted over and over again with new approaches, new products, and new ideas. The difference between a business owner and an entrepreneur is how they deliver that. We need to move forward, and we need to just say "yes".

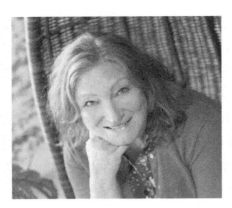

About Helen: You are a unique story. You connect with people through your smile, your physical presence, and your voice. What if you could do that online? Helen Snell is a storyteller, developing rich copy and content with personality. She connects your unique story to your prospect and your marketing strategy.

Your online profile and social media posts now represent the smile and handshake you used to offer at in-person meetings. Helen shows you how to use storytelling to make those connections. Adding key personal elements to your marketing through business stories lets people know who you are – not just what you do.

Helen's story process is used in developing biographies and profiles, web content, and marketing materials. She also provides ghostwriting for blogs and legacy stories. Her passion project is telling stories for the planet.

Connect your story with your client's needs and create a clear marketing strategy for your business through story.

76

BE SO POSITIVE PEOPLE THINK YOU'RE CRAZY.

REGINA BACZKOWSKA-POPELKA

hy: You should be so positive that people think you are crazy. Living a life of positivity is being happy. You have the time to travel and have new experiences. When you live a life filled with positivity, you have a genuine smile on your face. You can help people find joy in their own life. When you live like this, the bad vibes of others have no power over your life. This is not to say you won't have any struggles or hardships in your life, but you will have the strength and the habits to keep negativity and pessimism from gaining a hold on your life.

As a kid, I grew up hearing my grandmother's experiences during World War 2, and I will never forget those stories or how horrific they could be. And even though she had lived through so much, she always had a smile on her face, constantly reminding me that it could always be worse. I've learned now that this kind of positivity is not the kind of positivity that can push people to the next level of freedom and contentment with their life. Instead, it is the kind of positivity that sustains a person or a country when everything seems to have gone so wrong; it's survivor mode positivity. And that works too, but it is not where you want to be at all times.

But how do we make genuine positivity a habit in our life? Create an environment that will allow you to grow. To do that, you get rid of or limit the people or things in your life that bring out your negative thoughts and behaviors. And instead, find a healthy support group: tell the people that are close to you what you are trying to accomplish and ask for their support. Next, challenge yourself, start doing things that make you uncomfortable. Write out your whys. Write down what you are good at; write down one positive thing a day. Tell yourself every day that you are amazing, beautiful, and talented. Remind yourself every day that you are worth it because you are.

This year has been difficult for many of us in many different ways. But it is time to approach it differently; it's time to approach the world we live in with hope and positivity. If you positively approach your situation, you will have a different outcome. If that is really hard for you, start with the small things and every day try to one-up it. And one day you'll wake up and realize that positivity and hope are an hourly habit of yours.

HABIT

THE UN-HABIT: STOP DOUBTING YOURSELF

WHY: I have always been a positive and strong person, no matter what life threw my way. However, self-doubt was my kryptonite; it always prevented me from pursuing and achieving my dreams. I believe that this devastating cycle started for me when I was two, and my mom died. Then, once I was in school, I felt not good enough to have a mom because all the other kids had moms and not me. When I came to America at age twelve, I got bullied because I didn't speak English. I felt that the voice that told me I was not good enough was telling me the truth.

There are so many roadblocks to self-confidence in this life. We all have heard them. Some were told they were not pretty enough. Others were told that they weren't worth the time. Others were called stupid, foolish, or annoying, and their ideas sucked and to "forget about it" or "Be reasonable." Eventually, you find yourself scared, looking for approval in every direction, and unable to communicate your desires. It takes everything out of you to just believe that you deserve better, let alone stand up and make the boundaries that need to be made in order to live a healthy lifestyle. Just like that, life hijacks your self-confidence and leaves you with self-doubt.

But how on earth do I conquer my own self-doubt? To start, you have to set healthy boundaries. If you do not have good boundaries in your life, it invites other people to walk all over you. Poor boundaries leave you overwhelmed because you have more on your plate than a person is capable of handling. You end up in a cycle where all the important things are left either done halfway or not at all. Are you staying at work too much? Maybe you say yes to everybody even though you don't have the time to. Find the places in your life that are taking over it, and put parameters on them. If you're the person who always stays late at work, start leaving at your scheduled time. For those of you like me who always say yes, start saying no or the good old "I will need to check my schedule" or "I'm not sure I have time for that, I'll get back to you if I am available." It is better to say no when the alternative is feeling like you have no control over your life.

Next, what is your motivation? Some people will call this "Finding your Whys." These are the answers to the questions: why do you get up in the morning? Why do you want to be successful? What are your dreams? What do you want to achieve and why? You need to know these things because these are the reason you fight whatever lie of self-doubt throws at you this morning. For me, many of the answers to these questions involve or are my three kids. Why do you get up in the morning compared to lying in bed all day? I have three amazing kids that want and need me in their life, and I want to experience it with them. Why do you want to be successful? I want our life to be easier, and I want us to enjoy living it; I also want to be able to drop everything and go on a fancy vacation as a family.

This next one is the most direct at fighting your own self-doubt; Speak truth to the lies when they come. When the voice in your head tells you that you are not good enough, you have to fight it and, even more importantly, call it out as a lie. You have to actively recognize those doubts as lies, call them out on it and speak the truth back to yourself.

In conclusion, start fighting for the mindset that you want to have. Start fighting for the life you want to have. It is better to struggle towards the life you want than one day regret that you never went after your dreams.

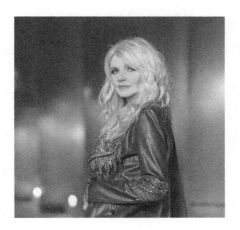

About Regina: Would you like to feel better? Healthier? Stronger? Yes?! Can I help you? I am a beauty health and wellness consultant. I have the most amazing products to help you take care of yourself from the inside out. Our products are vegan and cruelty-free. They also are soy, gluten, dairy-free, and so much more. Regina is also the creator of the SIMPLE Leadership Method™, which guides new, aspiring, and emerging leaders to become the leaders they would want to follow.

77

LISTEN DAILY
KAT MISCHE ELLE

Why: Start your new day by saying a mantra or prayer of, "I'm Listening".

This declaration for yourself should begin in your first phases of coherence when you first wake, shower, or when you are sipping on your morning octane beverage.

This sets the tone from within yourself to resolve all areas of your life where you may observe blocks that prevent you from moving clearly through.

By saying to yourself, "I'm listening", you will enhance and repair connectivity to your personal dynamics. You will increase being able to feel present in all areas of life, such as your career, romantic relationships, health, and wellness. This one habit creates and ignites positive productivity and counteracts that mundane or frustrating resistance lull you may be currently experiencing.

Commit to your 'listening' for an answer to present itself. It will arrive in a place, person, animals, time, event, the weather, or even an inanimate object catching your attention, and when you are "listening", it will be obvious to you.

With your declaration of "I'm listening", a daily habit of practice and application, you will hear a clear message of truth without the noise of words. Your listening will come from your full body of senses for what will be the best direction and/or choice to make.

This one habit will satisfy your life's current event's inquiries and the positioning of your next decision(s) on a regular basis. As your momentum grows, you will witness answers to be quick and true confirmations to the temporary challenge that presents its self.

The "I'm listening" habit is a time saver for indecisive individuals and busy professionals!

The "I'm listening" habit helps preserve your physical, emotional, and mental wellbeing. Tapping daily into "I'm Listening", will help to keep you sharp, focused, and in the steady flow of your life.

THE UN-HABIT: STOP SHOULD-ING ON YOURSELF

Why: Break one bad habit - "Stop should-ing on yourself".

(The word 'Should' refers to indicate obligation, duty, or correctness, typically when criticizing someone's actions. *definitions from Oxford Languages)

The emotional stressors of "should-ing on yourself" will only constrict the efficacy of your efforts.

Make sure you resonate with your tasks, instead, as a choice. Staying in a state of choice keeps you in your personal power, and when in your personal power, you will be in more of an emotional state of ease during your busy day of commitments.

While itemizing your upcoming tasks to complete, list them in order of importance, and then highlight the top three from that list. Once those top three are completed, then highlight the next top three most important from the remaining list. Continue this process until comments are finished.

Refrain from being frustrated with yourself if you cannot finish what you set out to do. That frustration is, "Should-ing on yourself".

If you perceived the day to fall short of what you set out to do, there is not a failure taking place! This correlates with the One Habit 'TO DO' of, "I'm listening." It is not a "No" to your efforts; it is just a "Not yet".

For example, to accomplish the tasks, your energy or mood may be better for the next day instead.

You may have been unknowingly in your own way the day before, so life positioned itself to set you up to win in a more productive way.... "I'm listening".

"Should-ing on yourself is on the shadow side of, "I'm listening".

Eliminate this one habit of "Should-ing" and you will see fewer and fewer obstructions, and you will start fulfilling your tasks with ease.

Refraining from "Should-ing" will not enhance a habit of non-accountability towards efforts or commitments.

By eliminating this habit of "Should-ing on yourself", you will only create more joy and efficacy where you choose to put your efforts for accomplishment.

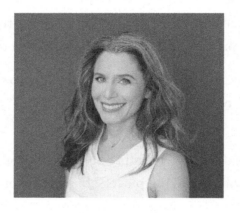

About Kat: Is an Intuitive Resolutions Expert who helps hard-working and fatigued individuals launch into the best versions of themselves through a perfected method of Quantum Voyance Integration.

Kat Mische Elle incorporates quantum physics, sociology, psychology, behavioral science, and alternative clairvoyance energy medicine to address and resolve challenges with anxiety, indecision, fatigue, and feelings of being emotionally constricted.

78

FIND YOUR ROCK

TRACY KING

Why: Getting into the habit of finding your ROCK is essential to creating desired life changes, especially after dynamic shifts in how we live and show up in the world occur. If change is what you truly seek, finding your ROCK must become your non-negotiable. That means uncovering whatever is hidden underneath it and making some decisions about what to do with issues and habits as they arise. To effectively do that, we must Release and Overcome what ails us, then Create and Keep what sustains us.

One day, Spirit led me down a path along the lakeshore. I came upon a developed area with huge boulders stacked like stadium stairs that probably spanned about a quarter mile or so. I was in a playful mood and envisioned myself walking a runway as the boulders served as my own personal cheering section. During my strut, I heard Spirit say, "Look for your rock." Ummmm, for real? I have a rock? I shrugged, "Okay, I guess I better find it then." I scanned the numerous rocks as I walked. They varied in color, size, and shape. Some were bigger than others. Some stood out because of their environmental imprint. I was not sure what I was looking for.

How would I know anyway? I kept walking until I came upon a rock I couldn't take my eyes off of. It did not seem all that special. I expected it to glow or something. Nope, it didn't. It just seemed to call me. I climbed about halfway up the pile to reach it. As I sat upon it, it unexpectedly shifted. "What the hell?" I thought I was going down. Immediately, Spirit chimed in... It may be a little scary, but I got you. I'm your rock. Solid. Strong. No matter what happens, no matter your fears, no matter how scary or uncertain your life gets, I've always got you. Your world may shift in unexpected ways, but I've always got you. I won't bend or break or let you fall, EVER. I've got you.

I sat in silence for a minute or two as Spirit continued to speak. I shed a few tears for a minute or two more. I was given some pretty amazing revelations on that beautiful day. I share this moment with you because I believe we all deserve to find our ROCK. Healing, growth, and manifestation occur for you when you do. So tell me, have you found your rock?

THE UN-HABIT: ROCK: RELEASE, OVERCOME, CREATE, KEEP

Why: As you identify, release, and replace "the old," you make space to embrace and engage "the new." The purpose of finding your ROCK is to stand on it and allow it to support you through the processes of life. Here's the kicker. Sometimes we carry our ROCK instead of stand on it. Why? Well, it's what we've been taught to do or what we've always done. Unfortunately, when you do anything but stand on your rock, its purpose is negated. It cannot support you. Instead, it siphons your power, energy, and focus. Imagine us all walking around bejeweled with ginormous boulders. I have mine draped around my waist, hanging down like an emblem on a chained belt. Yours is hanging around your neck as a charm. Wow, "I like that boulder; that's a nice boulder." Remember Donkey from Shrek? I am laughing just thinking about the scene when Donkey made a few negative comments about the surroundings they just walked into. Once he realized it was Shrek's home, he quickly changed his tune because he had a different agenda. He started complimenting the space instead, including those damn boulders.

It's funny how we do that in real life too. We can begin a conversation with a friend with all the best intentions and suddenly end up bitching, moaning, and groaning for hours about all kinds of nonsensical BS. We deep dive into the drama and negativity, complaining and co-signing the whole time. That's a lot of heavy shit and negative energy to put into the atmosphere. It's one thing to get things off your chest, but even then, we're spewing the undesired. Right? It is a whole other game, though, when you say what you need to say and keep feeding its negativity. Why fan the flames, which result in more of the same? You cannot manifest desires from barren places.

Your shoulders are not designed to bear that kind of weight. Please, do yourself a favor and put the damn boulder down. Stand on it instead. When you stand on your rock, you stand in and on your power. Anything that has previously thwarted, belittled, or victimized you are squashed by your rock and will forever reside underneath your feet. You see the whole world differently. It becomes yours for the claiming.

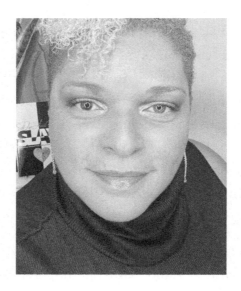

About Tracy: Tracy King, Life Midwife, Women's Health Nurse Practitioner, and #1 Best Selling Author.

With over 20 years in nursing, labor and delivery was and will always be my first love. That love catapulted my journey into Women's Health and beyond. Over time, it became clear that my desire to empower women extended far beyond the bedside. Now, as a Self-Love Expert and creator of the *SLAY (Self-Love Awaits You) Essentials,* I show women how to use self-love as a blueprint to live, love, and SLAY Life! By unlearning outdated modes of thought, you learn to inhale the magic of self-love and exhale all that has ever held you back. When you're ready to unleash the Goddess within, rebirth the life of your dreams, and experience the greatest romance that has never been told, come SLAY with me.

79

PUT YOUR FEET IN THEIR SHOES
JANELLE STRITE

Why: This 5 letter word changed everyone's world in 2020 - COVID. Some people lost jobs, and some people lost family or friends, some people lost their homes, some their minds, and still some lost hope. Regardless of what happened to you during the pandemic, we all endured some sort of experience in our life that probably shaped our opinion of the virus. And since everyone's perspective is different, it is super important to make a Habit of practicing empathy a part of your daily life when communicating with people about COVID-19. While I have had years of developing my empathy skills, it was not until coming out of lockdown that I realized the need to make it a Habit in everything I do or say to make clients feel comfortable in my salon. For the first time in years, my opinion did not really matter. What became a better Habit for me to do was to lean in and listen to each person's story or experience .... and believe me, we all have one. I then started learning from doing this with each client what was driving them to feel this way. Then I adapted my approach and speech to what made them most comfortable. I mastered it quickly because empathy is a skill... you really need to think about what people are saying. I gained from asking questions about their experiences the ability to quickly understand their motivations. I soon found using this mindfulness approach to people made a difference at work and in my personal life. I became more active in the here and now and what others were truly saying. I found it much easier to negotiate things, and it also became highly effective in conflict resolution. When I began teaching this Habit to other stylists, I noticed that managing my staff was increasingly easier as they were able to understand why I made decisions for the business, etc. But, alas, the greatest result we saw in this one HABIT called empathy was creating customer loyalty that no business owner can ever put a price tag on.

THE UN-HABIT: YES, YOU CAN SAY NO

Why: One Habit I would break is always saying yes. Exercising the power of saying no is an essential way of keeping your priorities in line. Stopping the insanity of trying to please others by always being the yes man can restore your own peace.

When you are saying no, you are honoring yourself and aligning your answers with your own values. I learned this new Habit also coming out of lockdown from Covid-19 (although we are truly not "out" of COVID yet).

I quickly found myself working seven days a week, somewhere between 15-18 hours a day. On day 22, I was on burnout. I was so close to the edge of losing my mind; I started developing migraines.

I now believe it was my body's way of telling me to slow down. I had to take a day off to handle myself. A whole day and I started panicking that I would upset my clients. While waiting for my shot of Toradol at my doctor's office, I learned my blood pressure was 179 over 100 and that I need to slow down. The only way to do this was to stop saying yes.

As I lay there waiting for the shot to kick in, a text came over my phone "any chance you can get me in this week" - it was the first time in forever that I said "NO". The reaction I expected was "ill try someone else" which meant for me lost revenue. The reaction I actually got was, "when is your next appointment then?" The next day, I set my hours, pricing, and goals for my business. If what I got asked did not align with those three things, I simply did not say yes anymore. At first, I cringed. I would lose clients, but it was not the case. Instead, what I gained by giving myself the respect I deserved was PEACE sweet PEACE. I got my personal life back, and it was all from breaking the Habit of saying "YES"

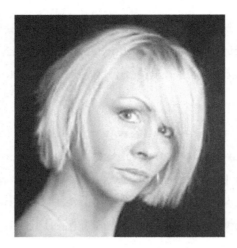

ABOUT JANELLE: Do you remember a time when you got into a dispute or a situation that you wish you could change? If I were to give you one to two things that you could do to change the outcome of those types of situations, would you be willing to walk and talk with me for a while?

80

KEEP MAKING CONNECTIONS
ALBERT COREY

Why: Do you know a guy that can help you with that? You likely would if you focus on being a connector.

You have to make the connections and become that Guy or Gal. It is your key to success in any environment. It doesn't matter if you are in a lockdown or a wide-open market. It's one section of your life that you can control.

In my world, I consider it a connection any time you have contact with someone. It could be as simple a liking someone's post on social media. Going to events and saying hi is another excellent way to let the world see you and connect to you.

The simplest way is to use what I call the power of free as your currency to meet other people. I have built a 7 figure business for almost four decades with this model.

It's a simple concept. Just go out to events or on summits and answer questions on whatever your specialty is without ever expecting any repository. You are not sending them to your Paypal link every time you open your mouth.

Share your knowledge and show you are the expert in your field. They might never use you, but you now "become the Guy/Gal" (who can help you with that). Funny how this phrase is your key to success. It might not show up overnight. It could take time before you start to see a payoff.

If you become the "I know a Guy" in a general conversation, you get the referral. The seed starts to grow when they run into you, and your expertise comes up. When you assist the first person and share what happened to another person, their friends will ask. Do you know anyone who knows about; (insert needed knowledge area)? Now your name comes up, and they say, "I Know a Guy/Gal."

The funny part of this it has worked since we have been keeping time.

THE UN-HABIT: GOVERNMENT MONEY MAKES YOU LAZY

Why: Some people have wasted hours trying to squeeze out a little extra money that the government will give out. They call us and ask if they have to pay tax on the unemployment checks.

Americans always find a way to move forward, so think for yourselves and pretend there is no government money coming, not now, not ever. Stop wasting time and get productive.

It is not the federal government's duty to give money out every time we hit speed bumps. The amounts are so small that it is not even a band-aid for your finances. Get productive; do something.

Shift your focus to success. What does that look like for you?

When you take your eye off the ball, bad things start to happen, like businesses shutting down, going out of business because of Covid. They do not know what to do, but others do. Shift and pivot!

Now more than ever, one must be laser-focused. The rich get richer because they always keep moving towards greatness.

We are seeing countless success stories of everyday people moving faster and making more money than ever. They are not sitting on their couch, watching TV.

Many people live their lives like it is the weekend seven days a week and watch Netflix just waiting for the government to take care of them.

But the knights in shining armour are finding other knights to band together with and move forward. They are not waiting for the government hand out. They're always on attack mode, knowing that they adapt or die.

People looking for the government handouts are shaking their heads, asking why the knights are moving faster than ever.

Walk into my office; the phones are ringing off the hook, all with people asking the same question. Where is my Stimulus

Check? (FYI The government has not even passed the bill yet.) Please find a better use of your time than worrying about where is your government check.

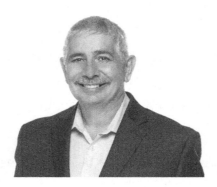

About Albert: He is known as the "Taxman." For almost 4-decades Albert and his staff at Corey and Associates have assisted over 16,000 business owners. Albert says, "let it rain money through simple marketing and accounting systems (that he affectionately)calls Nija Profit."

81

REMIND YOURSELF TO #BEPRESENT

KURT MILLER

Why: #BePresent -- This is my simple habit that has changed my life and will change yours too if you learn to use it.

Being a reformed workaholic (work in progress), I never noticed how my family saw me. I was there with them, but wasn't present, always thinking about work. Trips to Disney with my family, I would spend checking my phone and having text conversations while my body was on vacation. The entire time, I was oblivious to the reality that I was unfair to those I loved. Work was no exception. I was doing it at work as well. While in meetings, I would always be thinking about a dozen other things, having multiple text conversations with other people, and only giving partial attention to those in the meeting.

So in 2020, I discovered that a simple hashtag hack was all I needed. I remind myself to #BePresent. Two words. No deep internal discussions are arguments. Simply #BePresent. It has changed my life. Simply thinking to yourself, "#BePresent," and you will find that in 5 seconds, you can remove yourself from all distractions and focus on who you are with and why you are there. You can enjoy the precious life and time you have been blessed to spend with your loved ones. You can get more work accomplished during more productive meetings.

Most importantly, you can use #BePresent even when alone. Because we all need downtime, and #BePresent can be the tool you need to take time to go for a walk, work out, call a distant loved one, clean up the mess you've been ignoring. The list goes on and on.

So, in summary, I would challenge you to this. When in a 1:1 conversation or hanging on the sofa with a loved one (I am writing this while watching my 6-year-old play a Nintendo game), close the laptop, put away the phone, and #BePresent. You will not only change your life, but you will change theirs because people deserve your reciprocation of the attention they are giving you.

If you do this, you will find life has colors, smells, and joys that you have forgotten because of life's distractions. #BePresent my friend and live life.

THE UN-HABIT: FOCUS ON THE NEGATIVE

Why: #BeNegative -- Today's world has so many reasons to be negative. I am the living embodiment of #BeNegative. When I was 12, my parents decided to divorce and used me as a weapon against each other. This set my path towards being negative towards things and always protecting myself by looking for all the bad things in life.

Have you ever heard the term "Negative Nelly," "described as a frequently negative person? That was me. I would only see the negative side of things and focus on how everything is crumbling around me. I gave myself high blood pressure, super high anxiety. This affected my marriage, my career, and most of all, my life. I blamed others for this state of being because I did not have control of my happiness.

But after years of suffering the effects of being negative towards everything, I had an epiphany. The same energy that you use to be #BeNegative can be transformed to #BePositive.

You see, many years ago, I discovered negativity was simply a defense mechanism that I could put in place. Negativity became my shield, and by always embracing it, preventing opportunities. I reduced disappointment by anyone or anything, including myself.

Wow. Boy, was I wrong! I missed out on decades of happiness, all because of a child's insecurity that I continued to embrace throughout life. A simple shield put in place because of a trauma that wasn't even of my own making. And now I can see the light and color where I always saw darkness and gray. And you can too.

Simply break the cycle by flipping #BeNegative to #BePositive. Being negative or positive is simply a choice. It is not a physical barrier like a mountain that you cannot climb. It is a choice you can make. When faced with life's struggles, your choices are to stay negative or find a happy place that will bring a smile to your face and allow you to #BePositive.

When you feel sad, depressed, lonely, or the walls of anxiety are closing in on you, remember my words. As a matter of fact, I use Morgan Freeman's voice to hear "#BePositive". By using his voice, I shatter the walls of anxiety and let in the colors of the world instead of seeing the black and white negative vision. I challenge you to #BePositive and live life.

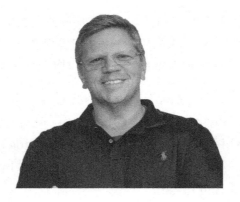

About Kurt: Have you noticed how so many companies work hard to get your business but then after getting your money, they #FailAfterTheSale? Whether you have a question about a process or the product fails to work as designed, you simply cannot get the time of day from their support team. I've heard horror stories of weeks going by without a reply.

Well, here at Support Made Simply, we've solved that problem. By leveraging decades of customer service, we have a system that will ensure that your customers don't feel the pain of

#FailAfterTheSale. Our technology prevents your customers from falling through the cracks of a support nightmare and instead will create a champion of your brand and someone that will want to buy your next offering without hesitation. Simply by flipping them from a negative experience to a positive experience.

82

NURTURE AND BE KIND TO OURSELVES.

SHERRY M HARRADENCE

Why: When we are in a Covid Pandemic like what we are in, we need to reach out, connect with others, and perform acts of kindness. It is such a wonderful feeling that makes you want to do more, and it is so personally rewarding and is a great new Habit to have. It triggers a chemical called oxytocin, which stimulates the brain with social connection and makes you feel good. We should all do something nice for our neighbors in need and set good Habits. Its contagious, and word will spread through out the neighborhood or community. Maybe taking a cooked meal to an elderly neighbor, doing light yard work, running an errand, get their mail, walking their dog, or doing some fun arts & crafts projects where everyone in the families may become involved. Whatever it might be, we need to help one another and unite our community as a whole. Remember, we are all in this pandemic together and need one another even after this pandemic. Our world needs a loving Global hug right now!

THE UN-HABIT: DOING EVERYTHING YOURSELF

Why: I hate it when someone says, "I can't do it," it's selfish. You need to replace it with yes, you can!! Believe in yourself. "I can't" prevents you from accomplishing your goals that you may have set for yourself. Remember, It's all in your outlook, mindset and you can do anything if you just try.

Habits are an act that repeat themselves without feeling or thinking. To break an un-Habit, you need to change your mindset to accomplish your goals and get control of your own power. Don't give up too easily...why lose and give away your power to something or someone else. You are strong, and with some will power to succeed and perseverance, you can do anything possible that you set your mind to. Let's replace those bad habits with new healthy and good ones.

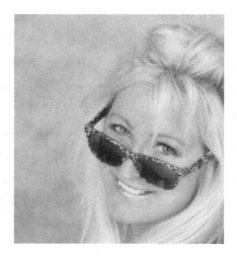

About Sherry: I am an artist who is a color addict and helps others express themselves by finding their creative voice through color and creativity. Art improves your health, mood, heals, and can make you feel much happier in your own space.

83

INNOVATE YOUR MARKETING

CARL RICHARDS

Why: We are living in a time where innovation is as crucial as pivoting. Businesses that have been able to shift during the pandemic have seen continued success. Are things different for them? Yes, in a lot of ways. That pivot or shift has been instrumental to their survival.

That can also be said of innovation, especially when it comes to marketing. What you did 15 years ago may not even apply today. What's different? Smartphones weren't a thing; Social media was in its infancy stages, podcasts were still in diapers. Heck, some businesses didn't even have websites! We still relied heavily on live events and more conventional means to communicate our ideas and market our businesses. Radio, TV, newspapers; they were all viable ways people got the word out. Imagine for a moment, if you will if your brand or business was still using a Yellow Page Ad. Likely you wouldn't be seen by many customers and would even have a hard time attracting new leads.

Innovation is how we will grow. People are online, period! People also want more 'proof' before they buy. Social proof, testimonials, Google reviews. Are you the real deal? That's what people are asking. They're also asking, 'how will you help me?' Which is quite different from, 'What are you going to sell me?'

As part of innovation, you'll need to provide that 'proof' (we call them touchpoints) over and over again—eighteen to twenty-four times. You'll need to stand out, be different, do what the competition isn't doing! You'll need to be in that category of ONE! Podcasting, for example, is a great way to do that. It's still very much the 'Wild West' when it comes to opportunity. Yes, more and more people are listening, and the number of podcasts is growing. There are still more blogs than podcasts, though, by a ratio of about 450:1.

If you want to be seen as the only option for business, the go-to expert, then do it with a podcast. It's a marketing tool designed to help you stand out on a global stage. Even if you serve a local market, people are adjudicating your services based on the market position. The business with a podcast stands a better fighting chance at visibility and exposure over the business that only has a website or blog...and certainly is light years ahead of brands still stuck on the conventional media conveyor belt.

The Un-Habit: Ditch tired thinking and beliefs

Why: Are you the same person you were yesterday? Some might argue, yes! I'm the same. Just a day older. Truly though, are you the same?

The answer is NO! You evolve every day. Or at least you should. How you show up, believe it or not, is in a constant state of change. Biologically we know this. We see it over time. In the physical sense, you're not the same person you were 20 years ago (even if you see yourself as young at heart). You've changed. Possibly gotten a few grey hairs or lost some.

Your thoughts need to evolve with you! What's unfortunate is, sometimes our thoughts grow in a non-fulfilling or non-productive way. They sometimes grow in a destructive way. Think of how full of energy and excitement to take on the world you were back 20 years ago. Are you just as excited to do so every day you wake up? Or has the world perhaps beaten you down a bit?

I can remember being so thrilled and excited to jump into my first career and rocket to the top, with little to no fear, full belief I could do this! When the wheel didn't go round a few times, I became a bit jaded. My thoughts and beliefs changed. What was 'possible' became 'impossible.'

In order to shift towards innovation, you have to once again think of what IS possible. The first thing that's possible is YOU and your success. Those old and tired beliefs need to go away, though. You need to shift your dialogue, make it positive, be fearless in your thoughts and beliefs. OR, become a part of 'what was.' For your marketing, it could mean being stuck with Yellow Page ads that don't serve you or your brand or being stuck with a dated website because you THOUGHT that's all you needed.

You need to reinvent and innovate almost daily. You're a new person every day. Your bad thoughts of yesterday, they're gone! Look ahead. Set your sights on what you want, push away old tired believe that keep you stuck. Allow yourself to truly be unique by embracing 'the new you' every day.

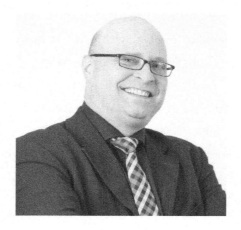

About Carl: Carl Richards has spent more than 20 years influencing audiences on stage and radio. The creator of Podcast Launch Made Simple.

Carl helps entrepreneurs and business professionals navigate the podcast world and showcases how to launch simply and with compelling content in 60 days or less!

84

MAXIMIZE BALANCE BETWEEN PHYSICAL AND VIRTUAL

LORI A. MCNEIL

Why: One important pivot to make in this post-Covid world we are changing and transitioning how we interact inside of our relationships, environments, and situations. Whereas before COVID-19, we were a physically engaged society, now we have become primarily virtual. We don't know just how long the virtual arena will be primary, and our beings were created to engage face to face. Here are some key strategies to help balance the physical and the virtual areas in life so that we do not lose the importance of our much-needed human bonding.

Certainly, the most physical interactions we will have are going to be with our families. Now, more than ever is the time to increase our communication with family so that those bonds are strong, the conflicts are less, and quality time is enhanced. This concept should permeate across all physical interactions we have... Maximize your time by quality.

The same goes inside our environments. Whatever physical space we find ourselves in, maximize its benefits. If you only have your yard, utilize it for your benefit. When you are at the grocery store or inside your office space, allow the permeation to infuse your environment as well. Maximize your surroundings by utilization.

Finally, whatever situation we find ourselves in physically, strive to be someone who engages others. Understanding where we are is important to engaging others appropriate for the situation. People are losing their ability to speak to others in the most mundane places, like the grocery store. Maximize your circumstances with presence.

Equally important is how we show up virtually. By now, we are all too familiar with the comedy concept of 'dressing from the waist up' while everything else is up in chaos. Before Covid, our virtual life was largely limited to engaging others who were distant. Now we could be having interactions with someone across the street solely virtual. Most of us have created a solid way to connect with others virtually.

What makes the virtual "acceptable" is leveraging it against the physical. Engaging in the physical builds strength, builds immunity, and breeds both empowerment and engagement, which positions us to be present inside the virtual. Remember to maximize your physical relationships, environments, and situations, and when you do, the virtual will feel more real.

HAB1T™

THE UN-HABIT: FEAR OVER FAITH

WHY: In everything that we do in life, there is often (if not always) a dichotomy between faith and fear. We should practice the art of acting with faith over fear. Too often, we operate with fear over faith mentality. No more present is this than right now.

When life becomes uncertain or when circumstances move beyond our control, our fight or flight system turns on, and we operate in 'safety mode' much like our computers (well, maybe just PC users) do when something attacks it. Pushing through and find the ability to develop a faith over the fear mindset and attitude no matter what is vital to removing the habit of fear over faith.

Our internal nervous system is set up to protect us, which is why it is easier to fall into fear over faith. Faith requires risk. Faith requires a journey into the unknown. Fear, on the other hand, requires us to stay inside of a comfort zone. Faith pushes us out of that comfort zone.

This is where breaking the Habit of thinking and operating from a fear mindset takes root. More than not, when someone labors from a place of fear, you will find unreasonable scarcity, unhealthy safety, and unbearable shock. These paralyze people from taking action that would push them through and beyond scarcity. Fear also creates a false sense of security by saying, 'don't take that risk' and forcing people to succumb to whatever is going on without fully embracing the situation to discover the truth. Fear also puts us into a form of shock, resulting in making bad or poor decisions or taking uncalculated and unstable risks.

If we can maneuver our thoughts from fear to faith, we can begin to see the world from a different angle. Distinguishing between fear and faith will help us make better choices and ultimately move us into a faith over fear perspective... across all areas of life. Faith over fear is power. Fear over faith is paralysis.

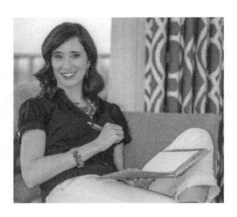

About Lori : Today's economy is so uncertain and unleveled that it is hard to know what to do especially when your foundation may not be secure. The key is - ensure you are aware of reality. Awareness creates accountability no matter what circumstance presents itself, and that accountability demands action. Lori has experienced incredible success leading her to focus on entrepreneurial success. From starting her first business at age nine to Media Secrets (her book and being featured in over 500 markets annually), coupled with her international speaking and business coaching, humanitarian projects (such as literacy, cancer research, and supporting our troops); Lori has become a force to be reckoned with. She regularly contributes to publications, has authored/co-authored several books, and co-founded "Celebrity U" which help entrepreneurs' level up their business. Lori will be launching this year her own business growth and legacy magazine.

85

BECOME YOUR OWN SUPERHERO
KEDMA OUGH

Why: I wish I could tell you that life plays out like a fairytale, but often, in our dire moments, we realize no one is coming to save us. We must learn to save ourselves. We must become our own Superheroes.

As the Small Business Superhero, I wear customized Superhero capes on stage. People often assume it is a gimmick or a costume until they learn the story behind the cape.

I wear the cape for two reasons. The first is never to forget; I am the hero of my own story. The second is always to remember to model heroism so that others can become the hero in their story.

Becoming my own Superhero saved my life. As young as 7, I remember praying to God to help me protect me and keep me out of harm's way. I would ask for guidance day after day, week after week, month after month, year after year. I never received it.

At the age of 18, my life changed forever. I was attending a community college in New York. While in an evening class, I received a 911 page from my therapist Judy. I remember grabbing my books and running outside towards the payphone. I dialed. "Judy, why did you page me?" She responded, "Listen to me carefully. He is on the way to the college. If he finds you, he will kill you. You need to get out of there". She was referring to my villain, and he was real.

I hung up the phone and went to the parking lot to search for my car. I was too late. He was there, waiting in his car, driving back and forth. Panic took over. I tried to scream, but I was in shock. My legs felt like quicksand. I thought, "Kedma, Run!" Yet, I couldn't run, as he would have seen me. I decided to crawl instead and crawled past each car to get to my car. I opened the car door, took my books, retraced my steps, and then called my partner for help. That would be the last time I would see my villain face-to-face. Overnight I became homeless.

I realized at that moment that no one was coming to save me. While there were people that cared, I had to save myself. I had to find a way to escape. I had to become the hero of my own movie. Today, I am still alive because I have learned that becoming your own Superhero could be the difference between life and death.

HAB1T™

THE UN-HABIT: RELYING ON OTHERS TO SAVE YOU

WHY: Once you break this Habit, you become the hero in your story. You stop waiting for others to come to rescue you. You stop blaming difficult circumstances that are in your way. You stop hoping for external forces to remedy your life. You no longer participate as an extra in your movie. You live out your life as the director of your movie. This allows you to choose the actors you want in your life scenes and puts the power play with you.

Even during my dire moments in life, as young as seven years old, I knew I was the hero in my story. While I couldn't escape the external trauma that I was experiencing daily – I still had power. I would sit in my closet and whisper over and over, "You can break my body, but you will never own my mind. You will never take away my smile or my ability to laugh". Even though I couldn't escape the circumstances, I still stood in my power and learned to use my mind to create imaginary experiences. My imagination always placed me in the hero position. I would close my eyes and pretend I was Wonder Woman. In fact, as I write this, tears are running down my face because I never stopped pretending I was the Wonder Woman in my life story.

Today, I embrace those images into real-life superhero work. I fight every day to help underserved, unrepresented businesses, and entrepreneurs access funding regardless of their financial circumstances. Even though I teach everyone the power of becoming a hero, I realize that we also need heroes surrounding us.

One of the most life-changing moments, representing this Habit's power was when I helped a disabled veteran apply for small business funding through the Veterans Administration. As a qualified business expert, I had reviewed and approved funding for the veteran. The agency denied him. I took on the case pro-bono and promised him that we would win the case. It took seven years, and we won the case. He asked, "Why did you fight for me for so long?" I responded, "because to ignore injustice is the same as creating injustice. I had no choice because it was the right thing to do. Now you can pay it forward with someone that will need your advocacy one day."

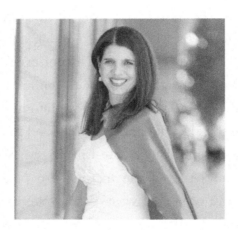

About Kedma: Kedma Ough, helps entrepreneurs, small businesses, and inventors find hidden funds to start, scale, and support their ideas and growth plan through alternative financing and grants. As a national expert in Target Funding, she helps create customized navigation funding maps so that the struggle to find capital is removed. Over 10,000 happy entrepreneurs have received a minimum of $ 10,000 in funding.

Whether you need $ 5,000 to launch your online store or $ 30 million to secure your government-funding contract, Ough can help. Areas of funding include equipment and vehicle purchases, real estate investing, business acquisitions, working capital funds, business grants, and licensing. Ough is also an accredited investor with Pipeline Angels and TBD Angels. Visit bit.ly/targetfunding for her bestselling book. Access to capital is one of the reasons businesses fail. It would help if you had a funding superhero in your corner. Ough also does keynote speaking engagements for major events.

86

START CELEBRATING
MEGAN HENRY

Why: Celebration activates and amplifies joy, which is one of the highest frequencies. Joy supports the expansion of life. I believe our purpose is to follow our greatest excitement and let our light guide us in every moment. When we are in celebration, we are in appreciation and in service to the highest potential for all.

As someone who was adopted, I felt a sense of guilt around my birth, which made celebrating birthdays feel somehow wrong. How can I feel good about my existence when my birth may have been a source of great heartache or disappointment for my birth parents? This disempowering story led me down an emotionally destructive path for years. I was incredibly jealous and didn't understand why other people got to feel good about themselves in celebration of their life and accomplishments.

The moment I started seeing my adoption as the gift that it is and started celebrating the opportunity to reclaim my power from my distorted perspective, my entire reality shifted. Instead of feeling I was given up, I leaned into the higher perspective that I was, in fact, wanted, so very loved, protected, and valued.

I invite you to lean into the idea that everything is an opportunity to step into higher potentials. What are your reality and emotional cues trying to show you? Everything is leading you towards greater self-realization.

Take jealousy, for example. You find yourself in a state of envy where you are witnessing a part of yourself, reflecting back to you in another, that wants fuller expression. Celebrate that awareness! Celebrate others' success because not only does it show you what is also possible for you, their success stirred up some discomfort so that you may know where you are holding yourself back. Celebrate that you can now give yourself permission to activate a part of yourself that you kept hidden.

There is a treasure in your triggers! Celebrate!

When you move through the world in celebration of who you are and able to see yourself as a gift—you are in service to your light. You become an example of the divinity you are, and from your beingness, encourage and inspire others to step into celebration, appreciation, and joy. You become love and higher consciousness in action. This new energetic paradigm supports our return to our natural state of abundance, joy, love, ease, flow, and unity consciousness.

A celebration journal is a great way to record the evidence of your successful treasure hunt and where you are expanding into more of YOU.

THE UN-HABIT: STOP COMPLAINING AND CRITICIZING

Why: Why choose to grumble when you can choose a grander perspective?

When you complain, you focus on that which you don't want and perpetuate the energetic frequency that contributes to the potency of the very thing you wish not to experience.

Bemoaning a situation immediately locks you into a fixed conclusion or story, that something is wrong. In higher states of consciousness, nothing is inherently good or bad. It simply IS. When you assign meaning to things, you limit your reality to even more significant and more satiating outcomes for yourself and another.

The discomfort you feel in situations is where there is a great treasure waiting to be revealed, and complaining dilutes the potency of the experience that is contributing to your expansion. When you stay loyal to complaining, you deny yourself the opportunity for deeper exploration of your shadow self and limiting beliefs. You miss the magical opportunity to alchemize your aggravation when blaming and criticizing yourself or someone else. Don't judge yourself. Shift perspective and your process.

While it is important to feel into your emotions and let the energy move to prevent stagnation and blockages, you can shift into a more neutral place of observation to the situation at play.

What if the situation at hand is really an opportunity to reclaim more of your power? To embrace your shadow self, heal, and alchemize? What if the relative that is triggering you is creating an opportunity to speak your truth or to set healthy boundaries for yourself finally?

When you are in a state of lamenting, you are giving your power away to perceived outside forces. You forget your connection to God/source energy and erode trust with yourself as the powerful co-creator within your reality. From this space, you miss the opportunity for expansion and grander possibilities. Moving out of criticism and into curiosity connects you to your heart center, your most powerful portal into impeccable creation/energy exchange. Start to infuse inquisitiveness and lofty questions into your experience. Rather than asking yourself, "Why is this happening to me?" Ask your higher self, knowing, "why is this happening for me?"

The answer may not come through immediately, and that's ok. This practice interrupts the pattern of complaining. Secondly, it also expands your energy into the field of possibilities and new ways of participating in your life. Lastly, it begins to calm your nervous system as it gives your mind the job of focusing on the solution.

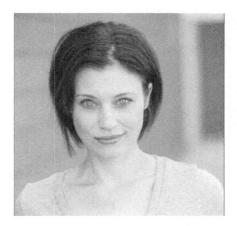

About Megan: You are meant to be seen, heard, and loved, in service to your gifts and your joy. Your greatest offering is your fullest expression as an aspect of the divine/god-source consciousness. You are here to remember. You are here to expand your greatest potential and the highest potentials for all life. Let go of complaints and criticisms and stand in your power. Get curious about your true essence and shine your light. Celebrate yourself, celebrate others, and everything in your reality, as it's serving in your expansion, no matter how uncomfortable. Where there is the most discomfort is where there is a great treasure to reclaim. When we give ourselves permission to look at what we are creating, we can see where we are either expanding or constricting our light. With tools to shift into compassionate curiosity, we can learn how to elevate ourselves into higher consciousness and love in action.

87

STAYING TRUE TO MYSELF
DANIELLE ROMAN

W hy: My lifelong belief is never to deviate away from your true self. When I was growing up, I remember whenever there was a situation that I did not feel comfortable with, if it did not match with my core values, I would walk away from it. My father taught us at an early age to be a leader, not a follower. We were always taught to observe a situation first and then decide if something worked for us. It is easy to be influenced at a young age into things that do not benefit us. I was always taught to be a leader, not a follower. At times, I found myself falling into the trap of people that did not have my best interest at heart. So, I had to learn from experience. The important thing is to learn from our mistakes. Fast forward to the Post-COVID-19 World we now live in. I understand this pandemic's seriousness, but I also understand we must make our own decisions based on our own personal beliefs. So, when I say "stay true to yourself," what I am essentially saying is, do not get sucked into all the hype and media frenzy and the opinions of others.

Ask yourself, Is what society and government asking of me in line with my core values and beliefs? Are wearing masks important? Sure. Is social distancing necessary? At times, yes. But at what cost? Am I being told to stay away from my family and friends? Are my personal and professional relationships suffering due to these rules and regulations being put upon us? To me, it is about controlling the masses, and I refuse to be a sheep and just follow. So, my friends, the one Habit I am committed to is staying true to my core family values and not allowing outside sources to control my life or steal my inner peace and JOY.

The Un-Habit: Wish I looked like a movie star

Why: Since I was a young child, I loved watching certain programs on TV and movies. I would always picture myself up on the screen as one of the beautiful actresses. They always looked so perfect, and I would think I wish I looked like them or wish I had a figure like that. I am sure many little girls like myself would fantasize about growing up and being an actress on the big screen. There is nothing wrong with "dreaming," but I had no idea at that young age of 9 or 10 the negative impact of comparing myself to others would have. It always took me to another world that was not my own but fiction. I felt empowered to envision myself in a different life than I was in. I guess I thought these famous people had a much better and glamorous life than I. In reality, they are just like you and me. It was not until I was a young adult that I began to understand the unnecessary pressure I had put on myself to be a certain way. I started on a path of not eating, extreme exercise, and not even running to the corner store without full hair and make-up. I was very self-conscious of my looks and weight to the point of obsession. And even though my family and friends would always tell me I am beautiful, that I do not even need make-up, and that I was at a healthy weight, my mind did not comprehend this or believe it. At that point, I was so convinced I needed to look a certain way no matter the cost. I walked down that destructive path for an awfully long time. It was not until I was literally in my 40's that I truly realized there was nothing wrong with me, I am not broken, and I do not need to be fixed. My husband and what he was teaching at his Spiritual Fitness Academy at the time we connected really opened my eyes to what I was missing all those years. I am already beautiful, inside and out, and I was made in God's eyes as perfect. When we compare ourselves to others, we insult our creator and ourselves as well. My father taught me a quote growing up. It says, "God puts us together, and we take us apart."

What that means is, we are born perfect, no matter what. We all try and find something to change and fix and add to ourselves, thinking it will make us more appealing to others. We are chipping away at our true value and just becoming something we are not. We find ourselves wanting liposuction, a facelift, a nose job, a straighter smile, curly hair, straight hair, whatever it is. Why do we working on getting ourselves further away from who we truly are instead of embracing what is right in front of us? I can honestly say I am finally comfortable in my own skin, and I genuinely love and embrace who I am today. Of course, I wish I had believed in myself a lot earlier in life, but I am also a big believer in everything happens for a reason. I was meant to go through everything I went through to become the amazing, strong, resilient, giving person I am today. I love to share my message with others to help them succeed. So, please do not compare yourself to others, especially to a realistically unattainable ideal. Love yourself for who you are, and remember, BE YOURSELF, after all... everyone else is taken.

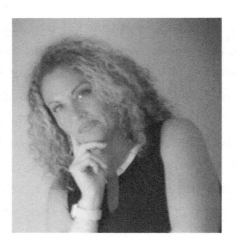

About Daniela: Daniela Roman created an online platform called Daniela's Delicious Dishes, which is directly in line with her and her husband's Spiritual Fitness Academy (An online Community of Fitness, Nutrition, and Spiritual Growth Tools) core values. What this entails is injecting the nutrition piece along with the physical and spiritual components of the Academy. Daniela has a passion for cooking and shares how healthy eating is so important not just to our physical well-being but also to our mental state. When we put healthy foods into our body, such as fresh fruits and vegetables and lean farm-raised meats, it influences our brain and thinking. So, when you lead a healthy lifestyle, it improves how you feel about yourself and improves your relationship with those around you. So enrolling in Daniela's Delicious Dishes course is the way to go if you want a simple "how to" of healthy meal plans set up according to your busy lifestyle. Daniela will show you step-by-step so you can stick to an easy get-up and go routine. When you look better, you feel better, and when you feel better, you perform better. They say, "Life shrinks or expands according to one's COURAGE." So in this New Year, have the courage to take that step and connect with Spiritual Fitness Academy and change your life!

88

REAFFIRM TO YOURSELF TO HAVE A PRODUCTIVE DAY

CATHERINE LAZURE

Why: When I was young, my mom used to tell me that there were "so many hours in the day," "time is of the essence," and "the early bird catches the worm." Another favorite was "winners never quit, and quitters never win." She never let me give up on anything academically or in sports and was my biggest cheering section.

When I was older, I realized what she meant by working; balancing family and community commitments took a lot of time. We need so many hours to sleep, work, self-care, reflect and dream, for family, and plan. My calendar suddenly became my bible, putting in everything I was supposed to accomplish, and by when, otherwise, I tended to waste my time, not have things done on time and let people down that know and love me. Worse, by saying "yes" all the time to asks for my time, I became burned out.

It's been proven that positive outlooks help for a more stress-free life and that affirmations are important to maintain a positive outlook toward ourselves and, therefore, be more productive. Creating a Habit to start each day with a positive affirmation of productivity helps us be accountable to ourselves and our busy calendars to accomplish what we set out each day.

With all the demands of our time and the distractions of cellphones and other electronic gadgets, we are easily distracted from our focus, taking precious minutes away from what might have been a productive day. One piece of advice aside from calendar blocking off time is to leave your phone in another room when you sit down to a particular task. If you're unable to hear the notifications going off and wondering who responded to your post, you can get more done.

The other big hint for productivity is learning to say no to all the tasks that come your way. As a humanitarian, I give a lot of my time to those in need, which makes me feel good to know that I am helping someone else who desperately needs it. Do what makes you happy, but within allowable time restrictions in adherence to your calendar & your health.

If you use your time wisely and efficiently, you will be able to free up some of your time for things you enjoy doing. Spending time with family, doing sports, fundraising for a favorite charity, or having that precious "downtime" for yourself are rewards for a productive day, month, and year.

HAB1T™

THE UN-HABIT: STOP WEARING TOO MANY HATS

WHY: As business owners, we have all heard the phrase "wearing many hats." Unfortunately, most make the mistake of trying to wear too many that don't fit their personality, their abilities, and their time constraints. If we are honest with ourselves, we are not great at everything. By drawing this conclusion and focusing on what you excel at, you can focus more time on doing things that will help bring up your productivity and business, as opposed to slow it down.

For example, suppose you are unfamiliar with how social media algorithms work and make posts. What are the best high-peak times to post on social media, the social platform's target audience, and how it pertains to your product or service? In that case, you could be spinning your wheels and losing a lot of precious time and money.

If you make your money by focusing on networking, client consultations, and fulfilling client needs, that is a better use of your time than spending it coming up with content, posting, and trying to engage on social media.

I learned this lesson as I was trying to build my website in the spring of 2019. I had made a few "cookie-cutter" websites but seemed to be at a loss with WordPress. Many tears and glasses of wine later, with many frustrating hours spent at my computer, I finally realized that I was wasting my time doing something that was beyond me, and it was time to get help.

Thankfully, I knew someone and have since added her to my team of VA's. Now I was free to go out, network, get our business out there in the marketplace, focus on our content, obtain and keep happy clients.

I make $30 per hour or more by doing work for a client, having had wasted at least 15 hours of not accomplishing anything on my website but frustration, it makes sense for me to take off the Website Developer Hat and pass it on to someone else better suited for the job. At the same time, I carry on facilitating my clients' needs. I make more with my clients than I pay a developer.

You can, too, make more money and have less stress. All you have to decide is which hat you're going to take off and let someone else wear.

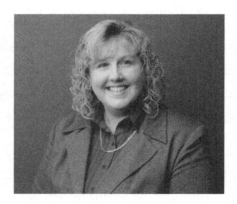

About Catherine: My name is Catherine Lazure, owner of CL Executive Solutions, a Virtual Assistant Company. We help small business owners claw back some of their time by doing tasks they either don't have time to do, don't want to do, or don't know how to facilitate their business. Our team specializes in a wide variety of areas that typically drain your time, including Administration, Marketing, Social Media, Project Management, Website Design, Development & Analytics, Bookkeeping, Event & Conference Management. We ask you to stop trying to wear all the hats and give us one or more you don't have time to wear so that you can focus on what you do best and maintain a work-life balance. When is it good for you to have a free 30-minute consultation to discuss how our team can help you take a hat off and claw back some of your time?

89

MAKE TODAY THE HAPPIEST DAY
LEE RICHTER

Why: Each morning, my daughter and I declare the following affirmations together "Today is the Happiest Day!" and "I Love My Life!."

In 2011, a happiness coach in San Francisco shared ideas with me to improve my happiness and to become more aware of habits that boost my happiness. At that time, I started incorporating daily affirmations to start my day in the best way. My daughter was seven years old at the time. I shared the daily affirmations with her, and at first, she was reluctant and asked a lot of questions. Over time, we made it fun, and we stuck with it —every day.

And now, almost a decade later, I see it as a beautiful way for us to connect and to elevate each other each day in a meaningful and positive way. We have made memes and printed photos to support this way of life. Powerful prompts help instill good habits!

Many of my friends have incorporated this idea into their life, and they tell me it makes an incredibly impactful difference. It's easy and free; start the day with a positive and intentional mindset, and you will see your day blossom into something special.

The Un-Habit: Stop being the victim

Why: When you want to eliminate destructive behaviors, I suggest you start by eliminating complaining! Complaining and seeing what is wrong tends to take people to a place of being victims and not to a place of empowerment. Besides, energy connects with like energy, so when you are complaining and seeing things negatively, that is the energy frequency you are attracting. And when you see things that are in a positive frequency, you will attract that more. So choose how to empower your brain and your day by choosing words and actions that take you closer to your goals and your best future self.

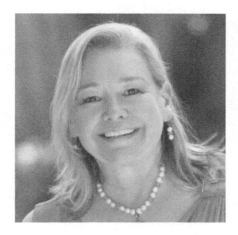

ABOUT LEE: Lee Richter is a business builder, best-selling author, speaker, mentor, and award-winning entrepreneur creating global brands in the technology, healthcare, and business world. Her expertise and business leadership helps teams and leaders succeed with a clear vision and plan.

90

DRINK TO YOUR HEALTH

TAMMY BOON

Why: It has been said that an apple a day will keep the doctor away. The new phrase in the 21st century is that a glass of water a day will keep the doctor away. Realistically that number of glasses per day is 6-12 and varies by the doctor advising the Habit. Confusing, right? Up to 70% of our body is water, which aids in body regulation and brain function. Humans can survive for days without food, but one day of inadequate water intake leads to the beginning of dehydration. The rule of thumb that I use to determine how much water is enough is simple: your daily intake in ounces of water should be half your weight (lbs). A straightforward way to determine what amount of water is adequate for healthy people and easy to keep track of throughout your day.

The most critical glass of water every day is the first glass that you drink. Yes, even before you have that first cup of coffee after

510 | 1 HABIT TO THRIVE IN A POST COVID WORLD

you have woken up, that glass of water is the most valuable one for your body. That first 8oz glass of water is needed by the body to immediately rehydrate it since you just went 6-8 hours with no water. The way that I look at it is this; I am watering my gut's garden, bringing it back to life.

I do my first glass of water differently than most. I add a ¼ teaspoon of baking soda to it, stir until clear, and drink. Why is this so important to me and my health? Covid was becoming known at the beginning of 2020, I was searching for ways to improve my health, so I would not become ill with it. I read research on an Alkaline diet because viruses do not survive well in an alkaline environment. I needed to know how to make my body more alkaline through diet because I knew my body was acidic, primarily due to my eating habits. By adding the 1/4 teaspoon of baking soda, I started my day with an alkaline body.

Then I found interesting information. I viewed documented interviews of the survivors of the 1918 Spanish Flu. The one thing that most had in common was their mom or grandma made them drink ¼ tsp baking soda in water every morning. Their families were the ones that never caught the Spanish Flu while taking care of other families that were ill with that contagious virus.

At the time of this writing, there is only one documented study with baking soda water, and the summary was that a daily dose of baking soda may help reduce the destruction of autoimmune diseases. I verified with my primary care provider that it was medically safe to drink ¼ tsp baking soda in water daily, and I started that regimen. I am an active person and working RN in daily contact with people that are Covid positive. I know I have been in close contact with contagious people, and I have not had one ill day since I added the baking soda water to my daily regimen of preventive supplementation. An ounce of prevention is worth a pound of cure. I am not giving medical advice, simply stating what I am doing for my health maintenance.

THE UN-HABIT: LACK OF HUMAN CONTACT

Why: One of the worst consequences of Covid and the ensuing lockdowns has been separation from those that we love. Not being able to travel to visit family or visit a loved one in a place like a skilled nursing facility or hospital are examples of that loss of contact. Extreme isolation from the societal restrictions and lockdowns are leading many to feelings of being alone, that there is no one there, and eventually to depression. A phone call does not give us that connection that we need to know that we are loved. Human beings are extremely social creatures, and we need contact; we need to know that we matter to someone, we need to know that we are loved, and we need to touch. Unfortunately, the Coronavirus pandemic is also causing a mental health crisis in America because of this extreme isolation leading to a rise in suicides and drug use.

Why is this connection so important to our bodies? The human connection contributes to healthy hormones and a stronger immune system, which we need in this post-Covid world.

How do we stay in contact with those that are loved and important to us? With so many social restrictions in place across America, it isn't easy. The answer is to use the tools that we have available in this digital age. Video applications, like Facetime, Zoom, and Skype, allow those that are separated to have a connection again, to be able to see and talk with their loved ones. Utilizing digital social applications allows people to be in touch with those that we love and care for. A fantastic way to let them know that we are thinking of them want to be in touch with them. It is not the same as being there in person, but seeing family and friends over the screen and talking to them like they are sitting there with you is rewarding.

The first Zoom that I set up for my dad (in Alabama) to visit with his sister (in Pennsylvania) was extraordinary. Watching them joke and tease each other, and them being able to see each other's expressions was priceless. They could not hug goodbye, but their bond was strengthened. Both of them were happier because of a Zoom meeting and could not wait to do it again.

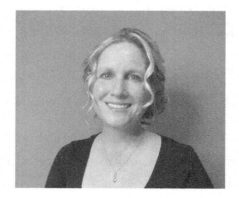

About Tammy: Tammy Mura Boon has been educating people about their health for 30 years. An ounce of prevention is worth a pound of cure so learn to think outside the box and dare to be healthier.

91

DO WHAT'S ESSENTIAL

SHARA HUTCHINSON

Why: "Start by doing what's necessary; then do what's possible, and suddenly you are doing the impossible."

~ Francis of Assisi

In March 2020, after confirming several new COVID-19 cases in Ohio, our Governor declared a state of emergency, followed by a series of shutdowns that appeared to be like a snowball effect. Public events were canceled, salons and schools were closed, childcare was limited, nursing homes banned visitors, restaurants couldn't offer dine-in options, and all establishments had a set number of people allowed to congregate. With so many businesses closing their doors in the interest of maintaining public health, there was one way to determine which would remain open: Businesses that were deemed "essential" because their product or service is a necessity for everyday living.

While all of this was taking place, I declared a "state of emergency" for myself. All my upcoming events were canceled, my plans were altered, supplies in the stores were limited, and childcare was not available. Although the day-to-day business had changed, my workload seemed to increase because all my worlds had collided. There was no work/life balance. Caring for a toddler while conducting meetings, leading a team, working on special projects, and juggling other home duties caused me to feel overwhelmed. Generally, I manage pressure well, but I felt like I could "break" if I didn't get a break. I was all over the place mentally, and although things around me had changed, I hadn't, and I hadn't changed for years. I was like the energizer bunny who kept going and going, going through the motions, going to unnecessary places, and getting involved in too many activities.

While those around me applauded my accomplishments, I knew deep down inside; I lacked focus. My attention was pointed everywhere and nowhere simultaneously. After feeling this way for about two months, I had an aha moment: Only activities deemed "essential" needed to get done. Coming to this conclusion was a game-changer. I felt more at peace, learned to be present with my family and friends, launched a business, published four books, started my podcast, had several virtual speaking engagements, and more, all in 6-months. I was able to do this by evaluating all activities and commitments by these 4 questions and then adjusting accordingly:

1. Does it have to be done?

2. Does it have to be done by me?

3. Does it align with my long-term goals?

4. Does it have to be done now?

I used the answer to question #4 for planning and scheduling purposes only. If the answer to 1-3 were all yes, I continued to do it. If one of those answers was a no, I ceased the activity. I even resigned from a board I had been serving on for four years because I realized it did not align with my long-term goals. It was a good thing, but not the right thing for me to do.

As you pivot in the post-Covid world, I encourage you not to go back to being busy just to be busy. Be intentional. Identify your long-term goals and then do what's essential to achieve them. If you start by doing what's necessary, then do what's possible, you'll find yourself accomplishing the impossible and experiencing sustained peace.

THE UN-HABIT: MULTITASKING WHILE WITH LOVED ONES

Why: "Multitasking: A polite way of telling someone you haven't heard a word they've said."

~Dave Crenshaw

"You never listen to me", my husband said, in the middle of a conversation because I could not repeat his last few sentences. I was on my iPad (researching business-related information) while simultaneously talking to him, and although I thought I could pay attention to both, I couldn't. I had no idea what he had just said, so there was no way I could repeat it. This further proved his point that I "never listen" to him. After seeing the sincerity in his eyes, I put my device down, looked at him, and then apologized for making him feel as if he wasn't a priority to me. I knew what he meant. I was in the habit of multitasking. Most of the time, when he sparked a conversation with me, I'd have one of my electronic devices in hand, "working" on something "important". I had trained myself to live in the future, working on goals while neglecting the "now". I had forgotten how to be present, and this was causing the man I love to feel unappreciated. At that moment, I committed that I would give him my undivided attention and not use any devices while we are talking.

"We are the generation capable of doing many things at once, without enjoying any of them."

Dinesh Kumar Biran

Several weeks later, I came across a blog that reinforced the importance of being present to me. In it, there was a story of a family. The wife asked her husband to take their children to school. The husband begrudgingly agreed to do it but made sure he expressed his frustration to her because he was already running late. As the father is driving with his children, he notices the traffic is slow and complains. The last straw was when they approached a railroad track at the perfect time to get stopped by a train. The dad was furious. Suddenly, his son said, "Daddy, we are so lucky. We get to see the train go by." While the dad felt inconvenienced, his son felt appreciative. They both saw the train going by, but one was frustrated while the other was excited. Perspective matters!

During the COVID-19 pandemic, I learned some precious lessons that revolutionized my perspective and enhanced my relationships:

1. Don't spend so much time building your career or business that you miss the opportunity to spend time building important relationships.

2. Slow down and designate intentional time for prayer and meditation.

3. Cherish every moment and always live on purpose.

4. Don't sweat the small stuff. If it won't matter ten years from now, it doesn't matter now.

As you pivot in this post-Covid world, don't multitask while spending time with loved ones. Give them your undivided attention and make good memories, not just good-looking pictures. Just as a global pandemic is unpredictable, so is every moment.

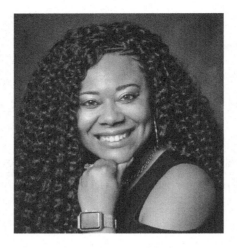

ABOUT SHARA: A TEDx speaker, Author of the Pebbles and Stones Planner, and Founder/CEO of Xposeyour; Shara has over 17 years' leadership experience and a proven track record of developing and implementing operational strategies and technologies that support key business initiatives. For organizations or leaders who want to boost staff productivity, improve employee engagement, stop making bad hiring decisions, or remove implicit biases from your interview process, Xposeyour provides services that help you develop a high performing team by getting the right people in the right seats and providing specific motivation for each individual. Unlike similar organizations, Xposeyour uses a science-based approach coupled with hands-on exposure to customized frameworks to align your organizations' people strategy with your business strategy. These services exponentially increase team cohesion by improving employee satisfaction and creating measurable results that ultimately impact the bottom line and enhance the overall customer experience.

92

AMIDST CHAOS, MAINTAIN MOTIVATION

ROBERT WALL

Why: Like a sailor pushing through a storm, you must maintain course, stay motivated, remember your training. Recall the fundamentals and skills that you acquired when the waters were still calm.

Here are a few proven methods for staying on course.

PASSION- When you do something you truly love, it's not hard to find the motivation required to succeed. If you are involved in an industry that bores you, it will be difficult to dig down deep and capture that motivation when you need it. You have to be truly passionate about what you are doing.

GOALS- I'm a big advocate of setting goals. Long-term goals give you something to work toward, and by including short-term goals, you're ensuring that you are able to seize victory consistently, providing further motivation to push hard toward achieving those long-term goals and visions.

Every single person is unique, and may prove multiple ways of staying on track; but over the years, I've witnessed a trend with highly successful people: Their goals are written down, and they have them accessible and review them daily. Whether in their face, like a whiteboard in their office, or on their phone with reminder alerts, or in that trusty notebook, successful individuals visualize goals, record, and take action on them.

BE OPTIMISTIC- When you are consistently optimistic, you focus on just the positives, which helps you stay motivated and focused on reaching your goals. The minute you start to bring negative thoughts into play, is the same moment your forward momentum will come to an abrupt halt.

Does the possibility of failure exist? Absolutely, but you cannot think this way. Entrepreneurs, visionaries, and leaders need to think like Olympic athletes. Do you think that for one moment a gold medal Olympian focused their mindset on losing every race? I'm willing to bet that the possibility of losing was still present, but they never allowed this to enter their mind. Their optimism dominated their thoughts, blocking out all negativity, and only focusing on the goal at hand.

These results won't happen all at once, but stay focused on YOU as the core brand—health, happiness, passion, purpose, and appreciation; you'll experience breakthroughs. Remain motivated in the hardest of times, and advance to a higher version of self.

Surround yourself with LIKEMINDED PEOPLE- This is probably the most important element. It has been proven that the company you surround yourself with directly influences how you behave, both in your personal life and in the workplace.

NEVER QUIT, because you've got this!

THE UN-HABIT: SAYING, I QUIT OR I CAN'T

Why: Simple, right? If you want to stay motivated and succeed, just don't give up. Not quitting gives you a 100% greater chance of success over giving up. However, plenty of people do, and the dreams they once had, become faded memories of could or should-haves. You can't possibly succeed when you stop moving forward. What if you continued to strive, though? Maybe, you would discover you were just a few steps away from victory. Imagine how grateful you'd feel if you could adopt staying power. You might have a dream you've thought about abandoning too. You'll never know whether you can turn it into reality unless you persevere.

Take small steps toward success if your dream seems too big and far from reach. Every inch forward moves you closer to your goal and helps maintain the habit of motivation. If you remain static, just thinking, instead of doing, you'll backslide and get nowhere. Be mindful; no step is too small to make a difference. Often, the actions you take to reach your dreams or goals, might be a series of tiny steps. Nonetheless, that minuscule shift can start momentum flowing, resulting in success and a more positive YOU.

Are your beliefs holding you back? There is an important connection between what you believe and what you do. If you believe "It's too hard for me to lose weight," "I'm not that smart," "I'm not athletic," "I'm a procrastinator," "I CAN'T"! Those fixed mindsets will cause you to avoid experiences of pain, failure, or to feel less-than. As a result, you'll lose motivation, missing out on the experience to learn from the mistakes that make you even better.

One of my favorite quotes "Whether you think you can or you can't, either way, you are right" – Henry Ford

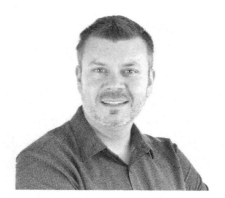

About Robert: Robert Max Wall - I help Executives, Entrepreneurs, and Small Business owners increase results through the power of Mindset and Self-Branding. Discovering who they are, the passion behind their offer, and to whom they want to serve.

93

DARE TO DREAM BIG
ANGELICA BENAVIDES

Why: Reasons you need to dare to dream big in life, especially during times of uncertainty.

Firstly, you need to dream big because you begin to set intentions in life that give you a sense of purpose. You will need to set intentions daily. What actions do you need to take to achieve your big dream? You will learn to monitor success. Are you getting closer or further away? Life is not just daring to dream big but taking the right actions.

Second is designing a road map towards your dreams. Where are you, and where do you want to be? It is vital to figure out the A-Z steps you need to take to achieve it. Designing your road map will help you gain awareness of the challenges and obstacles you might need to deal with during the process of achieving your goal to help you figure out who will help you through this process and what skills or resources you need to gain to support your dreams. The road map will clarify what new Habits you need to develop to accomplish your dreams; It will require you to evaluate what you do and how you do things in life. You will also have to evaluate your belief system. Many times, your belief system and current Habits don't support you to get to what you want to achieve. Your new

Habits will improve the quality of your life, and you will achieve your bigger dreams. As you work on achieving your big goals, you will also face more significant challenges, but you will develop resilience. You will also need to surround yourself with people who have achieved big dreams, which will move you beyond your comfort zone. To dream big and achieve big is to change behavior patterns, mindset, belief, plan of action, and network of people. Dreaming big leads you to expand your network, which will guide you to stay successful in your career and enhance your life quality.

THE UN-HABIT: STAY, FEARLESS

Why: It is time to stop playing small. We have been told so many times what to do in life that we wait for permission to Dare to Dream Big and Live a life we have no idea what it looks like or feels like, so instead, we go with the flow of the known. Now is the perfect time for you to claim your big dream because we are living a life of uncertainty. The world has experienced a significant shift; we have lost many lives and jobs and have been forced to do things differently, like using the virtual world more than ever. If you are ready to make 2021 your juiciest year yet, you will have to dream bigger and dare to take action towards what you want to achieve. Now is the perfect time to leverage and monetize your knowledge, experience, and passions for a more prosperous and juicier lifestyle.

I am supercharging my business as my big dream. I am spending more time clarifying who I am and what I want in business and life. I'd rather be rich, lit up while changing lives than being stuck in my old ways of doing things. I am okay with stretching beyond my comfort zone. I am taking fearless action, spending time using my imagination and visualization to clarify what I want to achieve in business and life. This step helps me explain my 2021 Vision that helps activate the Reticular Activating System (RAS). The RAS helps me pay attention and stay focused, prioritize, and focus on my heart desires. In other words, the RAS is in your brain that helps make goals happen. The most crucial Habit is to write down your goals to focus on what you want, which gives you a conscious direction to begin attracting people, things, places, situations, and opportunities into your life. You were born to be a leader and BE a high achiever.

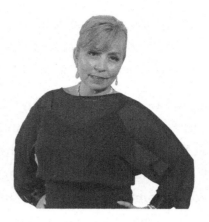

ABOUT ANGELICA: Hi my name is Angelica Benavides, and I am known as CEO Success Publisher and Business Strategist. I help entrepreneurs become World-Class StoryTellers & Best Selling Authors because there comes a moment in every person's life where you must make your presence felt, and your voice heard. Become Empowered and a Badass Influencer! Dr. Angelica is a visionary who believes in the power of expanding self-discovery and inspires entrepreneurs to reach greater personal freedom so they can help others do the same.

After being healed from two types of cancer, she knows she is here for a bigger purpose. She lost two of her homes, went through bankruptcy and divorce, but she broke through illness, financial hardship, and a broken heart by connecting to her Inner Divine Power. Now, she teaches everyone to tap into their Divine Power to achieve anything they desire. She inspires women to do everything in their power to live their highest potential. Her focus is to move entrepreneurs who are struggling to move from surviving to thriving mindset!

94

ESTABLISH AN OUTCOME BEFORE EVERY TASK

LAURA ARMSTRONG

Why: Time is so precious these days. We want to make the most of every minute, both personally and professionally. I was getting overwhelmed by family and friends trying to please others and say "yes" to too many things. I didn't want to disappoint anyone, most especially myself. I needed to make my life simpler, less complicated but still, feel like I was contributing to myself and others.

I have trained and taught Martial Arts for over 30 years and remembered that I got into the Habit of establishing an outcome before I would train or compete. I decided it was time to put this Habit back into my life. When I was competing, I would visualize and go over in my head what the outcome of the day would be. A first-place win for sure and envisioned how it would happen in detail, including receiving first prize. But most of all, it took the pressure off of any expectations I had because I had a plan and had planned out the outcome I was looking for. You may not always get the outcome you desire, but getting in the Habit to create one makes everything so much easier. Not only will establishing your outcome give you more focus, but it will also minimize the procrastination, distractions, and limitations we put on ourselves by not following through on things.

Our outcomes affect not only our business and leadership but also the personal aspects of our lives. They offer a clear plan and step by step process to success on all levels, and implementing this every time you have something that needs to get done; it can be as easy as saying - "When I buy a car today, I want to pay XXX and it has to have these extras." It can also help build your leadership as clarity in outcomes and what is expected is the key to getting people motivated and involved. They will want to follow someone who provides inspiration, a path to success, and the outcome of how to get there!

THE UN-HABIT: SETTING GOALS AND NOT FOLLOWING THROUGH

Why: Setting goals and not following through is like having bad New Year's resolutions: all words and no substance. It's disappointing and loads you up with all sorts of negative emotions that can have you spiraling downward, going nowhere. To continue to set goals you can't reach is unproductive and encourages you to procrastinate, leaving you in a negative mindset, thinking you can't do anything you put your mind to. Following shiny things without a plan will set you up for failure every time, fostering a sense of unworthiness, defeat, and incompetence. It's like complaining about something without offering a solution. It starts to get old, really quick. I remember it took me 4 World Competitions before I won a World Championship medal. I had to adjust how I set my goals, and the more I made them realistic and in alignment with my outcome, the better I got. And eventually, it paid off!! The more you start to set goals you can achieve, follow through on and accomplish, the better that will affect and ripple out to every area of your life. You will start to see that you do have the skills and tools to make things happen and effect change in your life on all levels. You can become the inspiration for others and realize that leading by example can be a way to grow your leadership and expand what you know and build your tribe. You will also find that your mindset shifts to a growth mindset where you are always learning and looking for ways to propel yourself forward.

Most importantly, you want to make your goals achievable. They have to be workable and realistic to what you need. Create a timeline and work back on it to make a plan where you can implement action steps to make it happen. Once you do, the sky's the limit!! So if you find yourself setting goals that aren't realistic, take a breath, reevaluate what you want, make a plan, and follow through!!

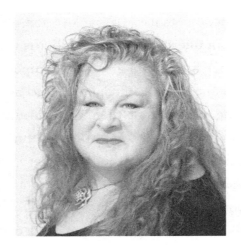

ABOUT LAURA: Leadership Accelerator - Communication Expert - As a 3X World Champion Martial Artist, I help you develop the skills, give you tools and map out the action plan to reach your full potential that will fast-track you on the road to extraordinary leadership success.

95

LOOK FOR THE GOOD

LESLEY KLEIN

Why: Look for the good: the opportunity in each situation, especially challenging ones. Ask the question, HOW can I? Instead of focusing on why you can't. When the "Great Pause" occurred, I was glued to the news to figure out what the heck was going on like most of us. After three weeks of this news diet, I became attracted to offers of free online webinars given by Raymond Aaron, Easier Life Online, Tony Robbins, Rise UP nation, and Forbes Riley. Many of these new thought leaders asked when "the Event" was over, where will you be? Fifteen pounds heavier? Or fit and fabulous? Thriving or just surviving? I took those questions to heart and decided to go down the positivity path instead of the path of the negative news black hole.

So I turned to the internet, not to focus on the negative news, but instead to focus on my personal growth and development. So 2020, for me, was a year of remarkable growth and productivity. I became a contributing author in an internationally best selling book. I started two online businesses and ended the year with creating a new talk show on the iSheTV channel featured on the SimulTV platform that reaches 182 countries!

I would have never have had these opportunities if I wasn't looking for the silver lining in the cloud of "The Event." As the phrase goes, when life gives you lemons, make lemonade!

So what information do you feed yourself? What are you focusing on? The first step is to be aware of where you put your attention. For, as Tony Robbins says: "where attention goes, energy flows."

The second step is to KNOW what you want. Forbes Riley challenged me with the question: "What do you want?" She has an effective method with the "what do you want" question to really dig down and find out what you REALLY want. I would love to introduce you to this superstar live during her Sunday Pitch Master Class.

Knowing what you want gives you the bull's eye to aim for it. And realize that you can change that bull's eye anytime! You are not married to it. The key is to make a DECISION and set a goal, realizing that that goal can be tweaked or changed at your discretion.

The third step is Forbes Riley's call to PLAY BIGGER. Playing bigger for me was a challenge because I was comfortable. My husband and I had retired and built a house in the North Carolina mountains. I didn't need to work; the basics were taken care of; however, I was bored at 57; I still had a second act, especially since I plan to live to a healthy 100. There was more to accomplish, and as "I was open to receive all my good" (Louise Hay). The Universe presented several opportunities to PLAY BIGGER, which included the chance to write a chapter in a bestselling book and an opportunity to host a television talk show!

THE UN-HABIT: HAVE TV NEWS ON 24/7

Why: We are so addicted to information these days. Our visual choices for news have grown from three major television network channels to hundreds of news outlets online, representing every perspective. Unfortunately, the news's thrust is negatively-oriented with a "blood and guts leads" news editor mentality. The outmoded way of thinking is to grab our attention with fear-based information. We watch the news and stress over a world we see spinning out of control with every calamity and disaster.

The physical reaction to such stressors puts us in the "flight-fight mode," After a while, we can become addicted to the adrenaline rush we get from being in a panic mode after watching the evening news. Don't you believe me? Stop watching the news. I dare you. And if you can't, try this experiment: limit your news intake (including social media news) to 5 minutes a day, so you stay current. Can you do it?

The real virus is Fear itself. Fear freezes us at its best and, at its worst, lowers our vibration so that our immune system is susceptible to whatever germ is at hand. It shrinks our creativity and causes us to play small. Fear is at the opposite end of the spectrum, with Love at the other end. Learn to raise your vibration to the Love and Gratitude frequency and watch your world transform.

Once you turn that external News noise OFF, notice the Peace that comes in to fill your world. Now you've created mental and emotional space focus your mental energy on your goals, on creating the life you want, regardless of what's going on in the world. Don't give in to Fear & Hate. Transmute it into Love and Gratitude. Be the Peace you want to see in the World!

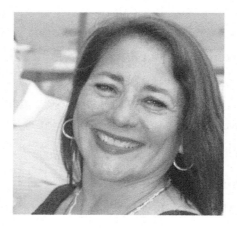

About Lesley: Lesley Klein has been an entrepreneur for over 26 years. Sixteen of those years, she created and operated an award-winning metaphysical bookstore in Florida. Her store specialized in personal growth and development, which helped her develop an eye for innovative products that up-level your life! The two life-changing products she shares with the world empowers you from your fingertips to your toes and everything in between.

Her business, Frequency Wellness Lifestyle, promotes the German-made Healy. It is a wearable wellness device that uses frequencies to balance & harmonize your four bodies (physical, mental, emotional, and spiritual). Her other business, Nailcraft, markets a fun, self-care product that raises your vibration differently through beautiful Do-It-Yourself manis and pedis using Color Street nail strips!

Her latest endeavor is producing & hosting a talk show called "Good-Vibes. TV," which will air on the iSheTV channel in early 2021. If you would like to be a guest or sponsor of her show, want a free remote Healy session, or a free sample of Color Street, find her contact on 1 Habit.com authors page.

96

SAY THANK YOU FOR THINGS THAT DON'T FEEL GOOD

NIKKI PRIVITERA

Why: From the time kids are able to mutter semi-coherent words, many parents are instructing them to say "Thank You" when given something that was desired. That something could be a toy for a birthday or a piece of candy. Sometimes they may even be instructed to say "Thank You" for a kind gesture. In fact, we as adults expect to receive a "Thank You" for these gifts and gestures and feel a bit slighted when it is not heard.

We have more recently been in the culture of gratitude. A good start for truly saying "Thank You," I might add. But in order to truly be grateful and receive the full benefit of that gratitude, it goes a lot deeper than being grateful for a safe, warm place to sleep.

When have you noticed the last time a parent instructed their child to say "Thank You" for falling and scraping a knee? When was the last time you expressed gratitude for missing out on what seemed like that perfect opportunity? For most, never.

In order to fully experience, I mean FULLY experience the wonderful things we experience, you must also truly be grateful for the less than wonderful things as well. Put this into perspective - would we understand if something was hot if we had never experienced something cold? Or, would we know if something was fun unless we also knew what was not fun? So how can we have gratitude for something we perceive as good unless we also know or have experienced something we perceive as not good? You see, we must also say "Thank You" for those not good experiences because they allow us to appreciate the good.

Often these "not good" experiences allow us to learn and grow. Napoleon Hill once said, "Every adversity, every failure, every heartache carries with it the seed of an equal or greater benefit." When we truly understand that every experience, every challenge, and every victory is deserving of a "Thank You," then we will truly experience the benefit of genuine gratitude.

THE UN-HABIT: PUTTING OTHERS FIRST

Why: When I was young and in vacation bible school, I learned a song called "Joy." "Jesus first. Yourself last. Others in between." Now, let me say that I am a Jesus lover, but I am not a lover of this song. Putting yourself last is certainly a huge disservice to you and everyone around you.

I am by no means implying to be selfish or self-centered. I AM implying to be self-nurturing.

I believe the author of the VBS Joy song was incorrect. I do believe the airline industry has it spot on. I am sure every single person who has ever taken a flight knows exactly what I am referring to. "If you are traveling with others or young children, secure your mask first, and then help others." In other words, make sure you are taking care of yourself enough to be in the condition to help others!

In our current society, many of us run ourselves ragged. We over-commit over-expect. And over-extend. We over empty. We attempt to maintain an unsustainable life. Often, it is an attempt to put others ahead of our own needs. We put the "needs of the business," the "needs of our boss to meet the needs of his boss, etc.," as a higher priority than the self-care that would enhance our ability to meet these needs more effectively. Or the "needs of our kids," which many times is the "need" to keep up with some crazy unsustainable activities.

What would it be like, what would YOU be like if we set healthy boundaries and you gave yourself some well-deserved love? Can you imagine having a restful sleep every night? What about your body feeling good or finding yourself having fun regularly? This can and should happen!

The simplest and most effective way to start is merely breathing. We already do this all day, every day. However, how you do it makes all the difference. Appreciate that every breath IN is a gift from the world around you. In turn, every breath

OUT is a gift you give back. We all learned this in 3rd grade, but the context was oxygen and carbon dioxide. When the perspective changes to receiving and giving, so does the breath. Try it!

Understand that by taking care and nurturing yourself, you can give so much more to others.

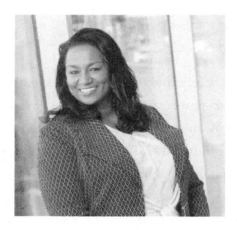

About Nikki: I support women in discovering and becoming their powerfully feminine selves in mind, body, and spirit.

A FEMININE WARRIOR is a woman who has recognized and accepted her divinely feminine traits to create and enhance her health, relationships, and purpose.

. . .

FEMININE POWER IS NOT about being feminist. It is about consciously embracing our natural health, beauty, resilience, intuition, and nurturing attributes.

THE ABILITY TO collaborate feminine wisdom and care with masculine power creates a Feminine Warrior and a more perfectly harmonized world.

97

STAY FIT AVOID THE COVID OBESITY

JANICE JAMAR

Why: Obesity has many pitfalls. It is uncomfortable to wear beautiful form-fitting clothing; obesity can also cause serious health issues.

Many individuals find comfort in eating their favorite foods. I, for example, have a weakness for potato chips and pizza. During my youth, I could plow through all sorts of junk food seven days a week. However, as I entered my sophomore year in college, I noticed that I couldn't overeat as before. The pounds began to creep up on my once athletic frame.

When COVID-19 hit the United States, it caused panic for many. Because of this, many turned to the bad Habit of munching fear and panic away. Not good, many have deemed this "pandemic weight" as an excuse to continue to overload on comfort food mindlessly.

Unfortunately, the snacking won't make the virus go away; it just adds another problem: unwanted pounds and lousy health. How do we stay in shape during a Post Covid World?

I like to call my remedy the 3 M's. The Memo, Mindset, Manifestation.

#1 Memo: Take a notebook dedicated to Staying Fit and write a memo each night before retiring. Write your goals for the next day. For example: "tomorrow, I commit to walking 30 minutes, no matter what. If the weather is inclement, I will walk inside my house!" "I will replace potato chips with sliced cucumbers and apples etc."

#2 Mindset: In your mind, visualize yourself successfully, having lost the number of pounds you have set forth to reach your goal. Your mindset is the fuel that will propel you to victory—Shun negative people. Surround yourself with individuals who have the same mindset that you have.

#3 Manifestation: To manifest is to make a vision in your mind come to fruition. See yourself already there; see yourself living what once was a vision, already in place. If necessary, cut out photos of fit bodies, and paste your head over the model's head. In your mind's eye, see this manifestation before you go to sleep and first thing in the morning. For reinforcement, look at it throughout the day.

Staying fit in a post COVID world is not a daunting task. Utilizing my three M's can get you on your way to cutting out bad habits, forming new ones, taking control of your appearance, and mitigating nasty health issues that obesity can cause!!! You can do this! I started it today. JOIN ME!

THE UN-HABIT: RID YOUR LIFE OF PESKY LITTLE CREATURES

Why: Procrastination is a pesky little creature that, if not caught and tamed, can ruin your life. It can lend itself to missed opportunities, destroying relationships, impeding promotions at work, lowering self-esteem, and being judged by outsiders gazing in and wondering 'why you can't get it together?"

It is important to break this Habit to live life more effectively. Manage the allotted time that each of us gets to live and participate successfully in life day by day.

This brings to mind, my Big mama. Big mama lived to be 100 years old. In Big mama's younger days, I always marvelled at how she structured her day. She was a self-taught person. When her feet hit the floor, she didn't get up from the bed and sit down, as many individuals do. Instead, she got up with her tasks in mind, and she accomplished them. It was then that she would relax and enjoy her favorite soap operas. She was not a procrastinator!

Although I marvelled at her efficiency, her Habit of getting things done did not rub off on me. I always gravitated towards putting things off until tomorrow or the next day, and if I could get away with it often, I wouldn't do it at all.

Herein lies the danger. In order to have a life that is efficiently managed there must be structure, there must be daily goals set, there must be time management. For some, like Big Mama, she had a knack for taking care of business until she finished. For others like me, tools are necessary to alleviate procrastination, especially when it affects living life and achieving goals successfully. Here are a few tools to use to keep procrastination at bay:

1. Prioritize tasks the night before in writing

2. Set specific goals and set a timeframe for completion of them

3. As goals are accomplished, strike them off of the list, then add another

4. Review the tasks each night, and make adjustments accordingly

5. Reward yourself as you complete your goals

Breaking the Habit of Procrastination is achievable. Taking baby steps is better than allowing it to take over, which will result in constant disappointment, low self-esteem, and missed opportunities. I plan to kick this Habit; I bought a notebook today, along with index cards, to get started. I won't stop until this Habit is no longer problematic in my life. Come on! Let's get started today!

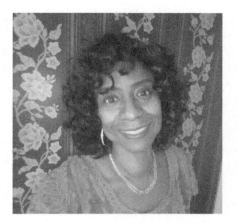

ABOUT JANICE: Everyone is focused on health, these days. A robust immune system is pertinent in guarding against all kinds of viral elements, seen and unseen. Although my products are holistic, herbal products, I cannot make medical claims, but I ask you to join me in sampling wonderful immune boosters, vitamins, detox teas, and CBD Products, to name a few! As a personal user of these fantastic products, my life has changed substantially. For example, the detox teas have a fringe benefit! Many have lost 5 lbs in 5 days. I am one of those individuals who have experienced this first hand. My favorite products are CBD products, which help with inflammation, pain, and anxiety. Try these products at my cost! I would love to hear your success stories, which I am sure that you will have when you witness the awesome benefits in your life, first hand!

98

TAKE STEPS TO MAKE YOUR HEALTH YOUR WEALTH

CHINEME NOKE

Why: Life as we knew it drastically changed for the whole World in 2020 due to the Covid19 pandemic (or plandemic). At the onset I was pontificating on, off and across social media as well as to anyone who would listen, that we must not panic; instead, we should assume that we are going to be infected with the dreaded virus so we must ensure that our immune systems are boosted so thoroughly that our bodies will see it off pretty sharpish.

Well, the trolling and ridicule that I received was astonishingly astounding! I had done my research and provided clear authorities and results of clinical studies which proved my point concerning the importance of our immune systems in fighting any type of disease, but the majority of my respondent's pooh-poohed the idea, laughed heartily at it and a good many were downright rude about it!

Undeterred, I continued with my recommendations of which Vitamins, Minerals, Compounds and Supplements that were recommended, as well as the appropriate whole foods we should be eating to strengthen our bodies from the inside. Some heeded my advice but largely, this was to no avail.

My knowledge around this area was highly developed after a car accident a few years prior had left me with post-traumatic, chronic, auto-immune conditions. Having always been into keep fit and good nutrition, I was astounded at the effects of the whiplash that I had sustained in my lumbar spine, as were a good many of the medical professionals that I encountered on my journey to seek a definitive diagnosis of what my body was so painfully going through. It took over a year to get some semblance of understanding, but it became clear that I was never going to fully recover. For a good few years I was virtually bedbound. This is when my quest for effective coping strategies began.

I researched and learned the function and real importance of our gut (intestines) and how we should be caring for it. I learned about the whole foods, vitamins, minerals and other compounds that were essential for good health – and I began taking them, as well as finding out the physical therapies that were also beneficial for good health.

I have now got to the point where I can engage fruitfully with the outside world again. I am able to be productive and creative, although I do still get debilitating flares when I overdo things (as I am wont to do!) I am in contact with others suffering with varying degrees of my conditions and, try as I might, it is difficult to convince people that there is a far more healthy alternative to the toxicity we ingest into our bodies for some slight relief (which are also immuno-suppressants).

Each to their own, but please do try to make a daily, conscious habit of consuming foods that boost, not compromise, your immune system – I've not had so much as a cold for many, many years and happily, a year on, the powers that be are now slowly but surely beginning to talk openly about the importance and supreme health benefits of boosting our immunity, naturally.

THE UN-HABIT: ABANDON ANY FORM OF SEDENTARY LIVING

Why: When Covid19 hit, lockdowns were mandated. This meant that the vast majority of people, who normally worked outside the home to make their living, had to stay indoors - together. They were forced to spend most of their time with their close family and relatives. Apparently, this produced a negative realisation for many couples that they were in fact less compatible than they previously believed in the good old days of necessary separation!

More importantly, many, many people began to suffer with depressive illness. Domestic abuse, suicides, and even murders were being frequently reported, said to be due to the fractious nature of being confined together in the home for extended periods of time. Such a situation had not been experienced by most people for many decades.

Enforced confinement was a shock to the human psyche, and with it came low mood, impolite behaviour and extremely sad emotions.

Hearing of these afflictions took me back to the horrific months and years following my post-traumatic, chronic conditions when I was virtually confined to my bed due to the intense pain and inflammation that I was experiencing. Due to my uncharacteristic, depressive state, my Doctor of 15 years referred me to a Psychologist who suggested that I do some gentle exercise, but I was aghast at the idea! Any small movement elicited yelps of pain and I almost believed that I would never leave my bedroom ever again.

Being a single mother and sole carer for my beautiful, teenage daughter with special needs, that of course was not an option. I began to write as a form of therapy. As my mind began to work again, I recalled one thing that Tony Robbins had mentioned that struck me when I saw him live so many years before. He said, "Your emotions are directly affected by motion." So, moving around can actually lift our spirits! With that reminder I pushed myself to get back to do some yoga, despite the pain.

Sure enough, as the weeks passed, I was also able to walk longer and longer distances, my mood began to lift, and I felt happy once more. I recalled my fit, energetic, unstoppable self and vowed to revisit her, albeit in a changed manner.

Therefore, such a valuable lesson (or reminder) was recalled – in order to achieve unstoppability in our lives, we must habitually get up and get our bodies moving!

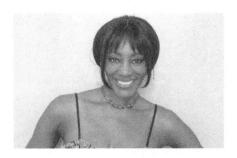

About Chineme: Chineme is a Corporate Lawyer, Success Coach, International Award-Winning, multiple Best-Selling Author of "Special Hidden Talents" and others, and an Online Entrepreneur. Her expertise is in all round Obstacle and Challenge Obliteration - with ease. She does this by dealing effectively with what she calls the mountains and molehills that success seekers encounter in their daily lives, by following her seven-step action plan formulated in her "Their Is No Time Like the Present to Create Your Future".

Chineme is the Founder of the Unstoppable Bizpreneurship program and the Unstoppable Shepreneurs private group. She is also the author of the soon to be published Unstoppable Shepreneurs: Become an Emboldened and Empowered Woman, Live an Exceptional Life and Leave Your Legacy."

99

TALK TO SOMEONE
MICHELINE ANNA SPENCER

Why: To get unstuck and moving forward in life.

Here is a story about two sports teams.

Team A and Team B both have injured players. If the players tell their coach about their injury, they will most likely have to sit out the season.

The injured players from Team A chose not to disclose their injury to the coach. Their coach did not understand why these players were not performing to his expectations.

The other injured players from Team B decided to tell their coach about their injury. The coach ensured the players received proper assistance from the team's doctor and the physiotherapists.

If you had to bet on one of these teams, which would it be? Why?

By not sharing the things that affect us, we get in the way of finding support. The people who care for us or groups or professionals won't have an opportunity to help. The players from Team B were able to play in the final games of the season because they had help and support to get them into top physical shape and ways to heal their injury. By not sharing our thoughts, emotions, feelings, we can hinder our ability to receive the support and encouragement we need. Living life in silence can cause us to think that we don't matter, or we are unnoticed, we don't belong, or we're unwanted. Beginning to make a new Habit of talking to someone about the situation can improve or change your life.

Changing your Habits is choosing to change.

Developing the Habit of talking to someone can feel daunting. More than ever, it is time to take a chance and talk to someone. As for the football players, there was a reason for being afraid, and yet they took action to share their injury with the coach, and in turn, the coach gave them the support they needed to recover. Sometimes sharing means we get "cheerleaders," someone who cheers us on, someone who has compassion, and most of all, someone who helps us move forward – get unstuck.

The Un-Habit: Stop keeping it to yourself

Why: Doing that will hinder you, not help you.

I had a good friend who encouraged me to share with my family about my struggles and my efforts. They said, "How can your family properly support you if you don't talk with them?"

This thought made me sad. Of course, I want help and assistance from the people who care for me. Keeping things to myself was an easy thing to do and very painful. And often, thoughts like "Don't share your problems." "Don't air your dirty laundry." "What can they do anyway?" would come to mind. I thought I was showing strength, but instead, I carried the pressure and weight of my struggles inside myself. So, I began to ask that critical question from my friend: How can my family or friend properly support me if I don't talk and share with them?

Keeping things to yourself (the good and the bad) can bring you down in life, especially when there are thoughts of feeling alone, feeling like you are the only one going through this, and no one will understand. The action to talk to somebody will open the door for assistance, relief, or just positive moral support. For example, an action to take might be finding a mastermind group, a fitness group, or a hobby class, which may provide you a way to a new world of help and encouragement that relates to you and your situation.

I have realized to make a Habit of talking to someone every day that there is usually hesitation. Therefore with just a bit of faith and trust, I go ahead and take that first step of reaching out to somebody, a friend, a coach, a family member, a self-help group, or a helpline. Over time and repetition, this new Habit provided the chance to feel heard, acknowledged, and stand for me. Sharing my truth, I now move forward in life with positivity. By taking the step to change my Habit, I changed my life.

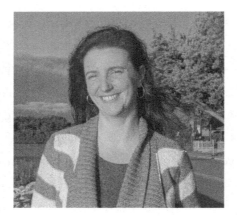

About Micheline: Blessed mother of 2 amazing young men, Kamal, a student in film and media, and Keynaan, a computer programming student. Teacher, Public Speaker, Author, businesswoman, and artist. Micheline has proudly worn many labels throughout her life. She has a degree from the International University of Hard Knocks. She's failed; she's succeeded. She's been married; she's been divorced. One of her biggest lessons is to share your truth, share your challenges with those you trust. Sharing who you are and what you are dealing with allows for your family, or friends, or community to become your biggest secret strength to help pull you through. Micheline learned that while keeping things close to your heart protects you at times, it can also create weight and sadness. One thing Micheline did to honor the lesson of sharing your truth was to write.

100

SAY THANK YOU FOR THINGS THAT DON'T FEEL GOOD

NIKKI PRIVITERA

Why: From the time kids are able to mutter semi-coherent words, many parents are instructing them to say "Thank You" when given something that was desired. That something could be a toy for a birthday or a piece of candy. Sometimes they may even be instructed to say "Thank You" for a kind gesture. In fact, we as adults expect to receive a "Thank You" for these gifts and gestures and feel a bit slighted when it is not heard.

We have more recently been in the culture of gratitude. A good start for truly saying "Thank You," I might add. But in order to truly be grateful and receive the full benefit of that gratitude, it goes a lot deeper than being grateful for a safe, warm place to sleep.

When have you noticed the last time a parent instructed their child to say "Thank You" for falling and scraping a knee? When was the last time you expressed gratitude for missing out on what seemed like that perfect opportunity? For most, never.

In order to fully experience, I mean FULLY experience the wonderful things we experience, you must also truly be grateful for the less than wonderful things as well. Put this into perspective - would we understand if something was hot if we had never experienced something cold? Or, would we know if something was fun unless we also knew what was not fun? So how can we have gratitude for something we perceive as good unless we also know or have experienced something we perceive as not good? You see, we must also say "Thank You" for those not good experiences because they allow us to appreciate the good.

Often these "not good" experiences allow us to learn and grow. Napoleon Hill once said, "Every adversity, every failure, every heartache carries with it the seed of an equal or greater benefit." When we truly understand that every experience, every challenge, and every victory is deserving of a "Thank You," then we will truly experience the benefit of genuine gratitude.

THE UN-HABIT: PUTTING OTHERS FIRST

Why: When I was young and in vacation bible school, I learned a song called "Joy." "Jesus first. Yourself last. Others in between." Now, let me say that I am a Jesus lover, but I am not a lover of this song. Putting yourself last is certainly a huge disservice to you and everyone around you.

I am by no means implying to be selfish or self-centered. I AM implying to be self-nurturing.

I believe the author of the VBS Joy song was incorrect. I do believe the airline industry has it spot on. I am sure every single person who has ever taken a flight knows exactly what I am referring to. "If you are traveling with others or young children, secure your mask first, and then help others." In other words, make sure you are taking care of yourself enough to be in the condition to help others!

In our current society, many of us run ourselves ragged. We over-commit over-expect. And over-extend. We over empty. We attempt to maintain an unsustainable life. Often, it is an attempt to put others ahead of our own needs. We put the "needs of the business," the "needs of our boss to meet the needs of his boss, etc.," as a higher priority than the self-care that would enhance our ability to meet these needs more effectively. Or the "needs of our kids," which many times is the "need" to keep up with some crazy unsustainable activities.

What would it be like, what would YOU be like if we set healthy boundaries and you gave yourself some well-deserved love? Can you imagine having a restful sleep every night? What about your body feeling good or finding yourself having fun regularly? This can and should happen!

The simplest and most effective way to start is merely breathing. We already do this all day, every day. However, how you do it makes all the difference. Appreciate that every breath IN is a gift from the world around you. In turn, every breath

OUT is a gift you give back. We all learned this in 3rd grade, but the context was oxygen and carbon dioxide. When the perspective changes to receiving and giving, so does the breath. Try it!

Understand that by taking care and nurturing yourself, you can give so much more to others.

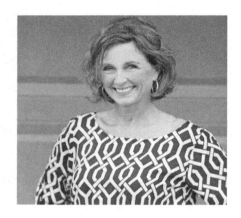

About Nikki: I support women in discovering and becoming their powerfully feminine selves in mind, body, and spirit.

A Feminine Warrior is a woman who has recognized and accepted her divinely feminine traits to create and enhance her health, relationships, and purpose.

Feminine power is not about being feminist. It is about consciously embracing our natural health, beauty, resilience, intuition, and nurturing attributes.

The ability to collaborate feminine wisdom and care with masculine power creates a Feminine Warrior and a more perfectly harmonized world.

101

CLOSE YOUR KITCHEN AT 6 PM
MAGGIE HUNTS

Why: Closing your kitchen after your supper will save you from the dreaded Covid 15, the 15 lb. that many people have put on.

Provide you and your family a balanced and nutritious supper with lots of vegetables and lean protein. When the dishes are all done, cut up a few veggies, and place them on the kitchen table for late-night snacks.

That is it; the kitchen is closed!

When you don't eat or nibble for eight or more hours, it changes how your body functions, and you start an intermittent fast. When you wake in the morning and eat your first meal of the day, what is it called? Break-Fast, you break the night long fast.

Intermittent fasting is helpful to our body and makes losing weight easy.

Make a fun barricade to keep your kitchen closed. It works!

THE UN-HABIT: NIBBLING ALL DAY AND NIGHT

Why: When you nibble all day and all night, you pack on the pounds.

When your body is receiving little bits of food all day and all night, it never goes into burning the fat mode; it just stores it.

You want to lift your spirits, not your blood sugar. Eating late at night raises your blood sugar levels and leads to weight gain.

Put the close the kitchen Habit into use in your home, and working at home can help you stay healthy, feel vibrant, and even lose weight!!

Eating all night fattens you up.

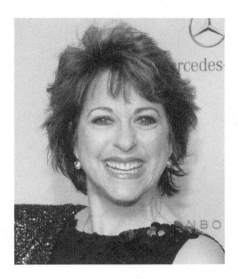

ABOUT MAGGIE: I've had type 1 diabetes for 35 years, and I HAD to solve eating to feel better. When I eat healthy fats, I'm not hungry; then it's easy to stop eating at night. I make it a game, and then it's fun and not a punishment. I have a three-story townhouse, with lots of stairs and I close up shop in the kitchen, and it works! No more food and no more unexpected weight gain. NICE!!! While working at home, food is always readily available, so don't buy sinful foods, and then you can't eat them. NICE! Lift your spirits, not your blood sugar, for healthy living and feel vital to work and live your contribution to the planet!!

102

WORK WITH OTHERS, PERSONALLY AND PROFESSIONALLY

JANE WARR

W hy: To thrive in a post-covid world, pivoting and changing how you do things is necessary. We live in unprecedented times, with "back to normal" not possible. Society and business don't go backward, but forwards, regardless of what they are going forward with or to.

At the time of this writing, we are several months into the pandemic that has changed how every single person communicates, personally and professionally. How we handle things emotionally, physically, and spiritually has changed.

We live in a society with family, friends, co-workers, and more. We are social animals, needing and thriving in community, benefiting from relationships with others. Now is the time to reach out to anyone, everyone, whoever can help you.

Asking for help or wanting help from others is not defeat. Let that go right now! That belief doesn't serve you.

Personally, connecting with others and accepting help leads to friendship, a sense of belonging, problem-solving, and more. Your self-respect, self-esteem, self-image, and self-projection will benefit. We each strive for happiness in life, which, as I see it, comes from having peace, love, and joy in our lives. Self-awareness is the start. Further knowledge of emotional intelligence includes self-management, social awareness, and relationship management.

Prioritizing relationships with self and others is critical now more than ever!

Professionally, relationships improve through everything mentioned above and more. Working with others can help you grow your network, market your products and services faster and farther, thereby growing your income and taking your business to higher levels.

You can motivate and inspire each other, have brainstorming sessions, form accountability partnerships, and improve skills. Promote each other's products, services, and events. You may choose to interview each other, start podcasts, co-host an event, or co-author a book!

A greater sense of community comes through business relationships too. Working with larger groups improves teamwork, morale, retention, and fun! The more people, and points of view, the greater potential for problem-solving, personal growth, improved skills, and leadership. Ultimately, we all strive to earn more in business while saving time, energy, and money; it is faster achieved with a team.

Make a list of like-minded individuals to contact. Know your objective. Are your businesses complementary? Know how you benefit them, how they may help you, and how others can be served as well. A win-win-win is always my suggestion, challenging times, or not! Be thoughtful during this period. Don't rush into anything too quickly.

"These challenging times" can bring out the best in us! By dropping your hesitancy to ask for help and raising your level of compassion to self and others, these can be exciting times!

UN-HABIT: THINKING YOU CAN DO IT ALL, ALONE

Why: Your Habits show you who you currently are; who you show up as, personally and professionally. The pandemic made our world far more virtual, with virtual gatherings, celebrations, business meetings, and events.

This isn't a time to try to be a superhero or prove something! This is a time to slow down to speed up. The entire world is affected, personally, and professionally. We all know people that have gotten sick have lost their jobs or incomes or worse.

Catch yourself having an egocentric moment, then challenge your thinking. How would working with another / others benefit you? Suspend judgment of yourself and replace it with grace. You can change your thinking within moments.

Many people were multitasking before the pandemic with work, kids, sports, and all that comes with it; they went into panic mode when the pandemic first affected them. Kids were going to school virtually, and adults worked from home, whether they had office space or internet bandwidth. Incomes were affected, and stress levels too.

Take each day, one day at a time. Check it to see what would bring more joy and fun into your life, not just less stress. I bet there are other people in that picture in your mind! Look for ways to save money, conserve and share resources with others. Think "big picture" regarding now and when "the new normal" is upon us.

Important: Get out of your comfort zone! You can not grow without reaching for new and different. Be open, allow, listen to others. Raise your level of respect for others and yourself.

You can choose to pivot, to restructure, to expand, and to receive. We are all a part of one global community; we commune and communicate with others to not just get through this, but grow, prosper, and succeed. Opportunities are everywhere. Seize them!

I believe in manifesting. We can manifest friendships, partnerships, collaborations, teamwork, and so much more. Stay positive. Energetically, put out what you are looking for with positivity and belief, and you will likely receive it.

Navigate the post-pandemic world by prioritizing your relationships personally and professionally. Apply the Habit of looking for others to work in conjunction with, and you will navigate the post-pandemic world with ease.

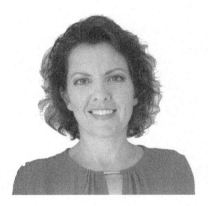

About JANE: Jane Warr, aka Trainer Jane, informs and inspires groups, as an award-winning Communications and Sales Trainer. She is a 4X International Best Selling Author and International Speaker, having shared stages with Forbes Riley, Loral Langemeier, John Shin, Bill Walsh and many more.

As the Founder & CEO of Selling on the Spot Marketplace; the #1 Networking, Sales Training and Marketplace, she provides fun and profitable events, serving the business community. She has taken the unique networking event company and built the brand globally through licensing and other collaborations. Other divisions include: Selling on the Spot Mastery, Selling on the Spot Marketing, Selling on the Spot Media Training (a partnership with Forbes Riley), Selling on the Spot Master Class and Selling on the Spot Systems too!

Her mission is to help YOU embrace the sales process, and sell ethically, efficiently and effectively!

ABOUT THE CREATOR OF THE 1 HABIT™ MOVEMENT

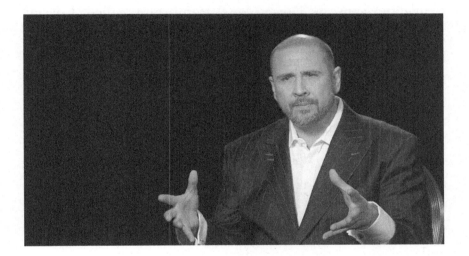

Steven Samblis is the creator of the 1 Habit book series.

He is the founder of 1 Habit Press. Before creating Samblis Press, Steven had a meteoric career in business that saw him go from being ranked among the top 50 rookie stockbrokers at Dean Witter, to speaking before 250,000 people for The Investors Institute. He has spoken before congress on shareholder's rights representing T Boone Pickens' "United Shares Holders Association."

In 1989 he founded "The Reason For My Success". which grew into one of the largest sellers of self-improvement programs in North America. The Company expanded into production where Steve collaborated with Chicken Soup for the Soul co-creator Mark Victor Hansen on the audio program The program, called "The Worlds Greatest Marketing Tools".

As a consultant, Steve created a new name brand for a struggling gym in Dover New Hampshire called Coastal Fitness. He then created a $9.95 a month business model which helped to turn the single gym into one of the most successful fitness franchises in the world, Planet Fitness. In November of 2015 Planet Fitness went public with a 1.6 billion dollar market valuation.

For six years, before launching 1 Habit Press, Steve was the on-air host and Editor in chief for Cinema Buzz, a website and syndicated television show in North America and the UK. On the show, Steve has interviewed over 1000 of the biggest actors and directors in entertainment one on one on camera.

facebook.com/samblis

instagram.com/samblis

amazon.com/author/samblis

ABOUT CO-AUTHOR - FORBES RILEY

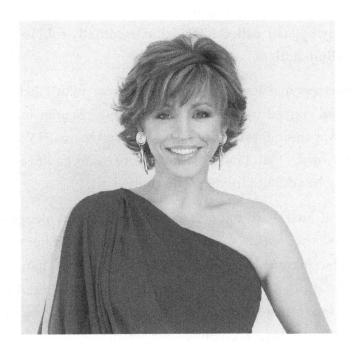

Starting her career as a Broadway, tv and film actress, Forbes gives new meaning to Renaissance women and striving for excellence in all that she pursues. Her doing stand-up led to a permanent hosting position at the Hollywood Laugh Factory working alongside Ellen DeGeneres, Jerry Seinfeld, Robin Williams and Wayan Bros. Her radio show career skyrocketed on Westwood One with the interview series Off The Record, getting raw and unscripted with Foreigner, Journey, Clapton, Steely Dan and more. When cable tv launched, her series ranged from the Dog Game Show Zig & Zig on Animal Planet, her own yearlong 2 women hosted talk show, Essentials on TLC, shows on Discovery, ABC Family, helping to create and launch the X-Games for ESPN (for 5 years) AND the launch-pad for selling fitness products on TV - the Hit 24 hour network with Body by Jake, called Fit-TV that eventually sold to Fox for $500 million dollars.

As an actress she has starred on Broadway with Christopher Reeve and starred in Lily Tomlin's Comedy, Search for Signs. Forbes appeared a variety of favorite Soap Operas, TV (24, Boy Meets World, The Practice) and more than a dozen films including her debut (Splatter University)

And as if that isn't enough career for several people, she pioneered the world of infomercials, alongside Shark Tank's Kevin Harrington, hosting and producing more than 200 of them and ultimately grossing more than $2.5 Billion dollars. A familiar face on late night tv, she won the hearts of America co-hosting alongside Jack Lalanne, Montel Williams, Mario Lopez, Bruce Jenner, Kim Kardashian, Tony Little, Betty White and P90x's Tony Horton to name a few.

When home shopping launched she worked for 28 years, not only QVC and HSN but globally at channels in Canada, Great Britain, Italy, France and Germany. Her key to success is her quick wit and mastery of the verbal art of communication and pitching. She now owns the Communication Arts Institute coaching and training entrepreneurs of all levels to perfect their pitch and monetize their messages both on and offline.

But wait, there's more. May sound cliché to some, but it's truly words that Forbes Riley lives by. In 2009, she elevated her game to a whole new level. After being inducted into the National Fitness Hall of Fame, she set out to create what many have called, the greatest fitness product on the planet. Her portable SpinGym is not only compact and portable so you get a resistance and cardio workout in anywhere and anytime but versatile enough to be used by bodybuilders and fitness competitors but people bound to wheelchairs, seniors, amputee, stroke victims and more. Her Dream Makers Foundation aids entrepreneurs from education to start-up funds and works with business on all levels to rise to their fullest potential.

www.Forbes360.com

www.PitchSecretsMasterClass.com

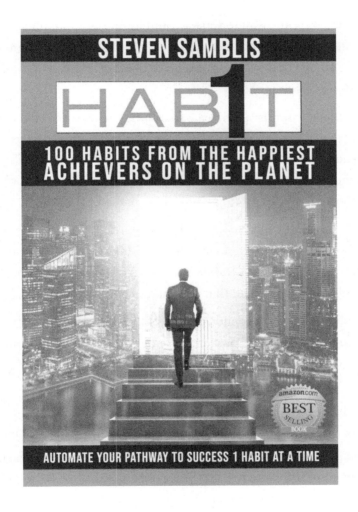

The Book That Started a Movement. 1 Habit™

You know the joy you feel when you are so passionate about your "why" that you can't wait to wake up and jump right into life? That motivation will get you started, but to be able to follow through, you need the Habits that will help you place one foot in front of the other when things get tough.

Author, Steve Samblis spent years searching the world for the most successful people on the planet. He got to know them and asked them each "What was the one most crucial Habit in your life that has made the most significant impact on your success." He then took these 100 Habits and put them into a book called 1 Habit.

Not only does the 1 Habit contain the Habits, but it also teaches you how to make a Habit part of who you are. Make it part of your being. Once instilled in you, the Habits becomes something you just automatically now do, and that automates your pathway to success.

Bottom line, you could spend 20 years of trial and error trying to find these Habits for yourself, or you can read 1 Habit and learn from others that have already done the work for you. 1 Habit compresses decades into days.

Lastly, the knowledge you will find in 1 Habit is not power. Execution is power. If you don't put these Habits into your life, what you have in your heart, your desires will honestly only be a dream. And, the last thing we want is for you to be 90 years old and you look back and say... "Wow, that was a nice dream." When it could be your reality if you start adopting these Habits into your life right today.

Get your copy at 1Habit.com/product/1-Habit/

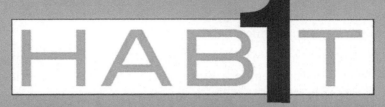
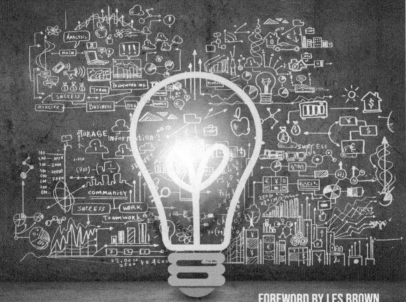

1 Habit For Entrepreneurial Success ™

What separates struggling small business owners from the powerfully rich? CEO's who seems to have everything working in their favor. They both embody Entrepreneurial Spirits, but one has superior HABITS. Little shifts from mindset to management skills can create stronger leadership, increased revenue, and ultimately serve a bigger impact.

To achieve unimaginable business success and financial wealth, you have to change your Habits to reach the upper echelons of Entrepreneurship.

You must develop a Positive Habitual Entrepreneur Mindset, a way of thinking that comes from learning the best Entrepreneurs' vital lessons.

1 Habit™ for Entrepreneurial Success brought together some of the greatest Entrepreneurial Minds on the Planet and asked them each two simple questions. What is the 1 Habit that has had the most significant impact on your life? What was the 1 un-Habit you needed to get rid of to clear your pathway to success? This book is the result, and the Magic is all you need is 1 Habit to change your life Forever!

Get your copy at www.1habit.com/product/entrepreneurial-success/

STEVEN SAMBLIS & LYNDA SUNSHINE WEST

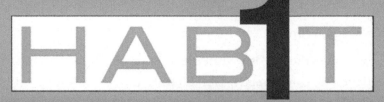

HAB1T

FOR WOMEN ACTION TAKERS

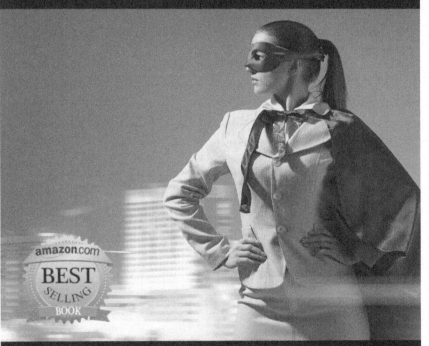

amazon.com
BEST
SELLING
BOOK

LIFE-CHANGING HABITS FROM
50 OF THE HAPPIEST ACHIEVING WOMEN ON THE PLANET

1 Habit for Women Action Takers ™

Habits Shape Who We Are.

The cool thing, though, is we can instill in ourselves good Habits. Even better, we can change bad Habits (aka un-Habits) into good Habits.

In this book, you will find stories from women action takers who are on a mission to make a significant impact on this planet by sharing their Habits and un-Habits to help you place one foot in front of the other when you need it most.

No matter how much you wish, hope, pray, desire, want, or manifest, nothing happens without action. You can see an opportunity staring you in the face, but if your Habit is to ignore that opportunity and turn the other way, that opportunity is lost forever.

1 Habit will challenge you to take an action step into the unknown. If you have a desire to be more, but don't know where to start, this is the book for you. 1 Habit For Women Action Takers offers small impactful steps that will help you create the life you have always dreamed of.

Get your copy at www.1Habit.com/product/wat

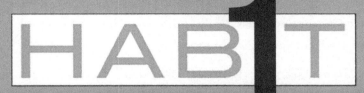

TO BEAT CANCER

FORWARDS BY
BRIAN TRACY & KATHLEEN O'KEEFE-KANAVOS

SECRETS FROM THE HAPPIEST CANCER THRIVERS ON THE PLANET

1 Habit to Beat Cancer™

Helping Cancer Suck Less: Daily Habits that Helped Incredible Cancer Thrivers Survive and Enjoy Life

1 Habit To Beat Cancer is a simple, easily digestible book that shares the new Habits that inspired these people to overcome their cancer as well as the bad Habits they did away with on their journey.

This book will teach you ways to overcome stress, feelings of despair, and overwhelm to feel instead determined and empowered to live your greatest life, and often, it takes JUST 1 Habit to change your life.

Get your copy at https://www.1Habit.com/product/1-Habit-to-beat-cancer

HAB1T

FOR SUCCESS...

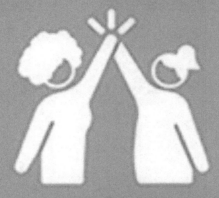

Created & Compiled by

STEVEN SAMBLIS

Co-Author **LEA WOODFORD**

FORWARD BY: LISA GUERRERO

SMARTFEM SUMMIT SPECIAL EDITION

1 Habit For Success - SmartFem Summit Special Edition

Imagine being mentored by some of the most respected people in the world. You are who you hang with, why not level up and learn from some of the most accomplished people of our time. This book will allow you to get an insider's look at the Habits of people who are on top of their game in all areas of these lives.

https://www.1Habit.com/product/success/

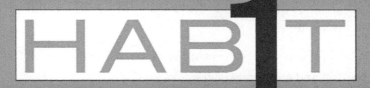

HAB1T

FOR CHRONIC DISORGANIZATION

CO-AUTHOR - REGINA F. LARK, PH.D.

LIFE-CHANGING HABITS TO END PHYSICAL & MENTAL DISORGANIZATION

There are common themes among the chronically disorganized that center around confusion and bewilderment about how effortless it seems for some people to get and stay organized, and how really, really hard it is for others.

This is how people start conversations with me <u>about</u> their disorganized and cluttered spaces:

- It's always been this way.
- I can't remember a time when...
- I've always been ashamed of this.

And chronically disorganized people tend to have a really lousy relationship with time, as in:

- I have no time
- I'm out of time
- There is no time

And there are consequences – minor ones (I forgot to buy the eggs!) and catastrophes (I'm late filing taxes again!). And all the consequences in between:

- High stress
- Everyone thinks you waste time
- Lose sight of personal/professional goals

1 Habit for Chronic Disorganization will give you the space to explore the chronic nature of this condition and how it lands in your life, and then help you unpack and dismantle its effects.

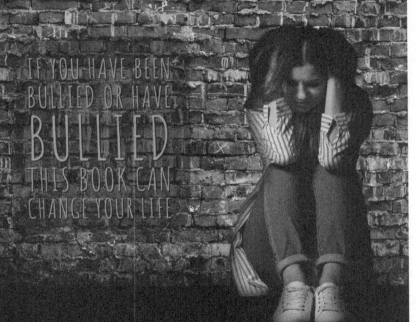

STEVEN SAMBLIS & KRYSTYLLE RICHARDSON

HAB1T

TO END BULLYING

IF YOU HAVE BEEN
BULLIED OR HAVE
BULLIED
THIS BOOK CAN
CHANGE YOUR LIFE

TOGETHER WE CREATE A BETTER WORLD

1 Habit to End Bullying

Bullying knows no barriers.

The dictionary states that the definition of resilience is the capacity to recover quickly from difficulties; toughness or the ability of a substance or object to spring back into shape; elasticity.

Resilience is needed in the case of bullying. It is true that bullying does not care whether you are a business executive, vice president of the United States, a diplomat of a foreign country, the cashier at a checkout counter, a high school baseball coach, Junior High School student or homeless person. There are people across all walks of life that have been affected by this poison.

https://www.1Habit.com/product/1-Habit-to-end-bullying/

ARE YOU A HAPPY ACHIEVER?

We refer to the Authors in the 1 Habit Book Series as "Happy Achievers." This is why...

For years, my life was focused on being a high achiever. Success was all I could think about. And success meant one thing and one thing only, how much money I made.

Throughout my journey, I would go out of my way to meet respected leaders in business, culture, and social change to learn their secrets and apply them to my success.

But, as I set out to create 1 Habit, I learned something even more amazing. It turns out, my desire to achieve was on target, but I measured it all wrong—in dollars and cents.

No matter how much money I made, I realized I wasn't as happy as I thought I'd be; there was always going to be someone making more.

One day it dawned on me, I needed to redefine what success meant to me. Money was not the right measurement of success. Money may be how others measure my success. Why should I give them this power?

I soon realized that happiness is how I wanted to measure my success. My happiness is something I am in control of. The way to reach happiness is to perform at your highest level in all plains of existence. The people that came together as contributors for 1 Habit all did this. These amazing people were all operating at the highest levels, Emotionally, Spiritual, their Physical Character, the way they live, and of course, financially. Happiness through the balance of performing and living at your peak in all those areas of their lives.

From that day forward, I would keep score based on the time I spent with my family, my friends, my hobbies, exploring the world, and realizing my passions and dreams.

I knew what I wanted to do now but did not know what to call this new category of a person that achieved highly at all levels and, as a result, were some of the happiest people on the planet.

Ask, and you shall receive

Whenever I have a question or a problem, I put it out there, and the universe always seems to give me the answers when I need them.

I was sitting with a friend who started out creating marketing campaigns for companies like ATT. He moved from there to head up a company that produces all major Hollywood studios' marketing campaigns. If you saw a movie in the last 20 years, there is a high likelihood that Mike Tankel was part of the reason you walked into that theater.

I told Mike about my new way of keeping score in life with happiness, not money. I no longer wanted to be a singular high achiever. I was something more. This thing was "the" more.

With little effort, it rolled off Mike's tongue. "You don't want to be a High Achiever. You want to be a "Happy Achiever". And there we have it. A "Happy Achiever."

So now I ask you, my dear reader. How do you keep score in life? More importantly, how do you *want* to keep score in life?

I hope you will join us and live your life to the fullest on all planes of existence. I hope you, too, will become a Happy Achiever!

Steven Samblis

Creator of 1 Habit™